Adult Nurse Practitioner Certification Study Question Book

EDITOR

Sally K. Miller, M.S., R.N.,C.S., C.R.N.P., C.C.R.N., A.N.P., G.N.P., A.C.N.P.
Vice-President
Health Leadership Associates, Inc.
Potomac, Maryland

Adjunct Lecturer
College of Nursing
Rutgers, the State University of New Jersey
Newark, New Jersey

Clinical Assistant Professor
School of Nursing
University of Medicine and Dentistry of New Jersey
Newark, New Jersey

Health Leadership Associates
Potomac, Maryland

Question Books

Family Nurse Practitioner Certification Study Question Set

(ISBN 1-878028-26-X)

by
Health Leadership Associates, Inc.

Consists of
The

**Adult Nurse Practitioner Certification
Study Question Book
ISBN 1-878028-20-0**

**Pediatric Nurse Practitioner Certification
Study Question Book
ISBN 1-878028-21-9**

**Women's Health Nurse Practitioner
Certification Study Question Book
ISBN 1-878028-22-7**

Additional Nursing Certification Study Question Books by Health Leadership Associates, Inc.

Acute Care Nurse Practitioner Certification Study Question Book
(ISBN# 1-878028-25-1), List Price $30.00

Adult Nurse Practitioner Certification Study Question Book
(ISBN# 1-878028-20-0), List Price $30.00

Pediatric Nurse Practitioner Certification Study Question Book
(ISBN# 1-878028-21-9), List Price $30.00

Women's Health Nurse Practitioner Certification Study Question Book
(ISBN# 1-878028-22-7), List Price $30.00

Family Nurse Practitioner Certification Study Question Book Set
(This shrink wrapped set consists of the Adult, Pediatric, and Women's Health Study Question Books).
(ISBN# 1-878028-26-X). List Price $60.00

Certification Review Books

Family Nurse Practitioner Set
(ISBN 1-878028-24-3)

by
Health Leadership Associates, Inc.

Consists of
The

**Adult Nurse Practitioner Certification
Review Guide
(3rd edition)**

**Pediatric Nurse Practitioner Certification
Review Guide
(3rd edition)**

**Women's Health Care Nurse Practitioner
Certification Review Guide**

Health Leadership Associates, Inc.
Managing Editor: Virginia Layng Millonig
                Mary A. Millonig
Production Manager: Martha M. Pounsberry
Editorial Assistants: Bridget M. Jones
                Cheryl C. Patterson
Cover and Design: Merrifield Graphics
Composition: Port City Press, Inc.
Design and Production: Port City Press, Inc.

Printed in the United States of America

Health Leadership Associates, Inc.
P.O. Box 59153
Potomac, Maryland 20859

Library of Congress Cataloging-in-Publication Data

Adult nurse practitioner certification study question book / editor,
  Sally K. Miller.
      p. cm. — (Family nurse practitioner certification study
question set)
    Includes bibliographical references.
    ISBN 1-878028-20-0 (pbk. : alk. paper)
    1. Primary nursing—Examinations Study guides.   2. Nurse
practitioners—Examinations Study guides.   I. Miller, Sally K.
II. Series.
    [DNLM: 1. Nurse Practitioners Examination Questions.   2. Nursing
Care Examination Questions.   WY 18.2 A2442 1999]
RT90.7.A38   1999
610.73'076—dc21
DNLM/DLC
for Library of Congress   99-22641
                                                               CIP

10 9 8 7 6 5 4 3 2

Contributing Authors

Sharon Fruh, Ph.D., R.N.,C.S., F.N.P.
Assistant Professor
Director Family Nurse Practitioner Program
Department of Community/Mental Health Nursing
College of Nursing
University of South Alabama
Mobile, Alabama

Carol Gemberling, M.N., R.N.,C.S., Ob/Gyn N.P., G.N.P., F.N.P.
Lecturer
School of Nursing
University of California, Los Angeles
Los Angeles, California

Cheryl Ahern-Lehmann, Ph.D.(c), R.N.,C.S., A.N.P.
Instructor
Nurse Practitioner Programs
Philip Y. Hahn School of Nursing
University of San Diego
San Diego, California

Reviewers

Preface

Health Leadership Associates is pleased to introduce one more component to our comple- ment of Nurse Practitioner Certification Review materials. This "Adult Nurse Practitioner Certification Study Question Book" will further assist the user of this book to be successful in the examination process. It should by no means be the only source used for preparation for the Adult or Family Nurse Practitioner Certification examinations. It has been developed primarily to enhance your test taking skills while also integrating the principles (becoming test-wise) of test taking found in the "Test Taking Strategies and Skills" chapter of the "Adult Nurse Practitioner Certification Review Guide" published by Health Leadership As- sociates. This review guide, in addition to the review courses and home study programs, pro- vides a comprehensive and total approach to success in the examination process. It enables the users of these materials to be successful in the test taking process and reinforces the knowledge base that is critical in the delivery of care in the practice setting. Many individu- als feel that taking practice test questions is the most important factor in the certification ex- amination preparation process, yet it is but one strategy to be used in combination with a strong knowledge base. Success in the certification examination area is based upon both ex- cellent test taking skills and a comprehensive understanding of the content of the examina- tion. As a nurse practitioner seeking certification, it is important to not lose sight of the defi- nition and purpose of certification. "Certification is a process by which nongovernmental agencies or associations confirm that an individual licensed to practice as a professional has met certain predetermined standards specified by that profession for specialty practice." Its purpose is to assure the public that an individual has mastered a body of knowledge and ac- quired skills in a particular specialty (ANA, 1979).

Inherent to the preparation for certification examinations is rigorous attention to the direc- tives and materials from the certification boards. Content outlines and sample test questions are often provided to examinees prior to the examinations. Specifics for each examination in- cluding suggested readings will be provided by the individual testing boards.

This question book has been prepared by board certified nurse practitioners. The questions have then been reviewed and critiqued by board certified nurse practitioners (content ex- perts) and a test construction specialist. There are 300 problem oriented certification board- type multiple choice questions which are divided according to content area (based upon test- ing board content outlines) with answers, rationales and a reference list. Every effort has been made to develop sample questions that are representative of the types of questions that may be found on the certification examinations, however, style and format of the examina- tion may differ. Engaging in the exercise of test taking, an understanding of test taking strat- egies and, knowledge in respective content areas can only lead to success.

CONTENTS

Health Promotion

Carol Gemberling

Select one best answer to the following questions.

1. The ANP has just completed a history and physical examination on a healthy 47-year-old accountant who has not seen a health care provider for over eight years. He has expressed an interest in becoming more physically active but is confused by all the recent information he has been hearing. Which of the following statements best reflects the National Institutes of Health recommendations?

   a. Research indicates that for the majority of people, exercise needs to be vigorous to have any beneficial effects
   b. The minimum standard of exercise for children and adults should be that they accumulate 30 or more minutes of moderate intensity physical activity most days or daily
   c. The health benefits of physical activity can only be obtained if an individual exercises three times per week with intensity at 60% to 85% maximum heart rate
   d. To be effective, exercise requires an initial level of fitness, skill, special equipment, and uninterrupted time

2. One of the principle objectives of the U.S. Preventive Services Task Force project includes which of the following?

   a. Preventive services, which are tailored to meet the individual needs of the patient, have been proven to be effective in properly conducted studies
   b. Guidelines for preventive services are mandated for all health care providers to use in their clinical practices
   c. The project's objectives supersede other task force recommendations for the management of patient problems
   d. The task force's key objective was to keep the spiraling cost of health care within reason and prevent overuse of the health care system

3. Mr. Elmore is a 68-year-old African-American client who presents for an annual examination. His problems include borderline hypertension and asymptomatic carotid artery stenosis. He has not had any recent laboratory or diagnostic testing since his annual examination one year ago. Which of the following laboratory tests are indicated as part of the cost effective preventive care for this otherwise healthy and active client?

    a. Hepatitis series and carotid ultrasound
    b. CBC and Hgb A_{1c}
    c. Fecal occult blood testing and lipid panel
    d. Chemistry panel and diphtheria tetanus

4. Mr. Cummings, a 52-year-old asymptomatic client, has a 30-pack-year history of smoking cigarettes between the ages of 15 and 45. His history and physical examination are unremarkable except for the fact that he is concerned about lung cancer, because one of his army buddies recently died of lung cancer. He wants to know if there is a test that can be performed to diagnose lung cancer since he smoked for so many years. Which of the following statements best reflects current thinking?

    a. Sputum cytology is a helpful diagnostic modality
    b. Routine chest radiography should be considered
    c. Bronchoscopy would provide the necessary information
    d. There are no mass screening tests available for early detection

5. Mrs. Bartwick is a 54-year-old opera singer who has visited your busy family practice for her routine women's health care for several years. She complains of mild flatulence and rare bouts of diarrhea which she associates with the daily ingestion of caffeinated sodas. She denies a family history or personal history of bowel diseases or cancer. Which statement best reflects the current thinking regarding preventive health care for this client?

    a. Based on her symptoms, a digital rectal examination is the diagnostic procedure of choice
    b. Based on her age, a digital rectal examination, fecal occult blood testing, and sigmoidoscopy are the procedures of choice
    c. Based upon her age and her symptoms, a colonoscopy is the procedure of choice
    d. Based upon her symptoms, a barium enema is the most cost effective diagnostic modality

6. While performing a pre-employment history and physical examination on a newly hired telephone cable installer, you detect alcohol on his breath. During

the brief occupationally related history, your client states that he rarely drinks more than a beer or two on the weekend. His physical examination, including Romberg and coordination testing, are within normal limits. Which of the following actions is the most appropriate response?

a. Assume that he was so delighted to finally get a job, that he probably celebrated over lunch with a drink
b. Perform a blood alcohol test even though it is not a routine part of the assessment for new employees from this company
c. Perform a CAGE test to screen for a possible drinking problem
d. Immediately refer him to an employee assistance program so that his problem can be assessed and managed confidentially

7. Ms. Rupert is a 23-year-old patient being seen for second trimester prenatal care. This was an unplanned pregnancy and she reports feeling irritable, which alternates with listlessness and insomnia. She has developed a dry cough and hoarse voice but denies any upper respiratory symptoms. Her partner is concerned about her behavior and called the office before her visit because he is concerned that there is something wrong with her. Recently she has begun socializing with her old friends again. Her physical examination is unremarkable except for harsh breath sounds over the parasternal area. Her fundal height is 20 cm, and her LMP was 22 weeks ago. Fetal movement was noted. What is the next step you would take in the management of this patient?

a. Inform the patient and her partner that it is common in the second trimester to have feelings of irritability and listlessness
b. As a part of today's evaluation, assess for a history of behavioral problems or drug abuse
c. Counsel the partner that it is normal for her to want to be with her friends and that the insomnia will disappear in the third trimester
d. Consider referring her to high risk obstetrical care after consultation with the supervising physician

8. Mrs. Palmer is a 51-year-old mother of three who comes to you for a breast examination, after thinking she felt a lump about two months ago when she first learned to perform breast self examination. She can not find it today, but is still concerned about breast cancer because her great aunt had breast cancer diagnosed when she was 80-years-old. Mrs. Palmer reports that she has never had a mammogram because her breasts are always so tender. Today, the visual inspection and palpation of the breast, axilla, supraclavicular and infraclavicular

lymph nodes are normal. No masses were palpated although bilateral, symmetrically distributed mild tenderness was noted. Based upon your evaluation of this patient, the next appropriate step would be to:

    a. Inform her that her examination is normal today and that she should return to see you in one year for another clinical breast examination

    b. Refer her for a screening mammogram, review breast self examination, and advise her to return in one month for a follow-up visit

    c. Suggest that she have a diagnostic mammogram and an ultrasound

    d. Refer her to a breast center because her family history puts her in a high risk group and she is in need of closer evaluation

9. Mr. McDermott is a 72-year-old gentleman who has recently relocated to the United States from England following the recent death of his wife. His diet consists largely of fast food, and he has stopped the daily walks he used to take with his wife. His son brought him to the clinic today for the third measurement of his blood pressure which has been elevated. When he was in England, he took some medicine every day but his little yellow pills were lost in the move. Today's blood pressure is 162/92 mm Hg, which is comparable to the other two readings recorded at previous visits. Which additional information is required before the ANP can establish the most appropriate management plan?

    a. Discuss whether or not he will be compliant with his management regime

    b. Assess his willingness to enroll in a group with other individuals who have recently lost a spouse as this might help reduce his blood pressure

    c. Begin the diagnostic evaluation for causes of secondary hypertension including pheochromocytoma and renal artery stenosis

    d. Assess for additional cardiovascular risk factors and presence of any target organ diseases

10. Mr. Sanchez, a 58-year-old architect, has come into your office for a discussion of the results of his physical examination and laboratory tests. While discussing the results, he questions you about the health of his prostate gland and wonders why you did not order the blood test he has heard all of his friends talk about. In light of the controversy and risk benefit analysis that presently exists, which of the following statements best reflects current thinking regarding prostate screening tests and their usefulness in low risk patients?

    a. The test that he heard about has too many false negatives to be clinically useful

    b. Evaluation of the prostate with a prostate specific antigen test is performed yearly in all susceptible men

   c. Since prostate cancer is among the top three killers of American men, it is important to obtain a prostate specific antigen test

   d. Routine screening for prostate cancer with digital rectal examination, serum tumor markers, or transrectal ultrasound is not recommended

11. Mrs. Davis has returned for re-evaluation of her knee pain which has improved in the last three months. She is greater than 40% above her ideal body weight and has been working hard to keep off the 23 pounds she lost last year. She has been able to maintain her low calorie and low fat nutritious diet and feels that the exercise bike and walking are easier for her to do on a regular basis. She tells you that she understands that high blood pressure and diabetes are more common in "heavy" women, and recently she has heard that she might also be at risk for certain types of cancer even though she has a negative family history. What would be your best response to this patient?

   a. Cancer of the breast, colon, cervix, ovary, and endometrium are increased as obesity increases

   b. Cancer of the throat, melanoma, thyroid, and brain are increased as obesity increases

   c. Cancer incidence increases in the testicle, ovary, colon, and rectum as obesity increases

   d. Cancer incidence is not increased in association with obesity and that she is at the same risk of developing cancer as the general population

12. As a new ANP you have just begun working in a student health service as a nurse practitioner. Your patient, a 25-year-old female graduate student, does not know where her immunization record is, and needs to bring her immunizations up to date before the semester begins. She is certain that she has not had any immunizations for over 10 years. Her history and physical examination are normal and there are no contraindications to receiving immunizations. Which of the following immunizations would you consider giving her today?

   a. MMR, PPD, hepatitis series and DPT

   b. Rubella vaccine, coccidioidomycosis skin test, PPD, and Td

   c. None without her immunization record

   d. In rubella negative individuals, MMR, PPD, and Td

13. During a part time position as a nurse practitioner, you begin working in an upper class neighborhood in California. While being oriented to your position, you notice that neither the staff or other health care providers are asking any questions to assess patients' risk for injury or violence. At the end of your first day, as you review the day's events, you ask the physician why this part of the

history is not addressed. You are told that in this population of patients, it is extremely rare to find any type of domestic violence or abuse. Which of the following statements best reflects current recommendations for providers?

a. In settings where the prevalence of violence is high, clinicians should ask about previous violent behavior or victimization, current alcohol and drug use, and the availability of handguns or other firearms
b. Every client needs to be carefully assessed because despite the lack of evidence that the client may be a victim of violence, providers need to be suspicious that abuse may exist
c. The presence of firearms in the home is the key indicator that the potential for abuse exists, and a thorough assessment should be performed to rule out the potential for violence acts
d. A comprehensive assessment should be performed on all of the adult clients in this population, but adolescents and youths are not as vulnerable to crimes of violence

14. Which of the following is recommended as minimum preventive health services according to the *U.S. Guide to Clinical Preventive Services?*

a. Pneumococcal vaccine for all healthy persons over the age of 50 years
b. Annual influenza for healthy individuals starting at age 65 years
c. Colorectal cancer screening for all healthy people over the age of 35 years
d. Cholesterol screening beginning at the age of 18 years

Answers and Rationale

1. **(b)** The NIH has defined physical activity as "bodily movement produced by skeletal muscles that requires energy expenditure and produces progressive healthy benefits." Very sedentary people will benefit from any increase in activity (Patem, pp. 402-407).

2. **(a)** The report of the U.S. Preventive Services Task Force was intended to guide health professionals in the judicious and cost effective use of preventive services that are individualized by both age group and personal or family history (USPS Task Force, p. xxv-xxxiv).

3. **(c)** The U.S. Preventive Services Task Force has recommended that persons age 65 to 75 with risk factors such as smoking, diabetes, or hypertension should be considered for cholesterol screening (USPS Task Force, table 4).

4. **(d)** Routine screening for lung cancer with chest radiography or sputum cytology in asymptomatic persons is not recommended. There are no large scale early screening programs available at this time. The best advice is to counsel all patients against tobacco use (USPS Task Force, pp. 135-139).

5. **(b)** Screening for colorectal cancer is recommended for all persons aged 50 and older with annual fecal occult blood testing, or sigmoidoscopy (periodicity unspecified), or both. Insufficient evidence exists to determine which of these screening methods is preferable, or if the combination produces greater benefits than either alone. The American Cancer Society recommends routine screening with the digital rectal examination. Based upon the U.S. Preventive Services Task Force Guidelines, there is insufficient evidence to recommend for or against routine screening with digital rectal examination, barium enema, or colonoscopy, although recommendations against such screening in average risk persons may be made on other grounds. Persons with a family history of hereditary syndromes associated with a high colon cancer should be referred for diagnosis and management (USPS Task Force, pp. 89-99).

6. **(c)** Screening to detect problem drinking is recommended for all adults and adolescent patients. Screening should involve a careful history of alcohol use and/or the use of standardized screening questionnaires. Routine measures of biochemical markers is not recommended in asymptomatic persons. All

persons who use alcohol should be counseled about the dangers of operating a motor vehicle or performing other potentially dangerous activities after drinking alcohol (USPS Task Force, pp. 567-578).

7. **(b)** Standardized questionnaires or biological assays performed routinely lack sufficient evidence of efficacy when it comes to suspicion of drug abuse. All pregnant women should be advised of the potential adverse effects of drug use on the development of the fetus. Being alert to signs and symptoms of abuse in patients, and referral of drug abusing patients to specialized treatment centers, is the most important role that practicing clinicians can play in the war against drugs (USPS Task Force, pp. 583-591).

8. **(b)** Women aged 50 to 69 should have routine screening for breast cancer every 1 to 2 years with mammography and annual clinical breast examination. There is insufficient evidence to recommend for or against the use of screening CBE alone or the teaching and reinforcing of breast self-examination. The American Cancer Society supports the teaching and reinforcing of BSE as part of a program of breast health. The number of lumps that women detect in their own breasts warrants consideration of continuing to teach and reinforce BSE as a standard of care (USPS Task Force, p. 73-84).

9. **(d)** After the diagnosis of hypertension is confirmed, patients should receive appropriate counseling regarding physical activity, weight reduction, dietary sodium intake, and alcohol consumption. Evidence should be sought for other cardiovascular risk factors such as elevated serum cholesterol, smoking, diabetes, obesity, peripheral vascular disease or target organ damage (USPS Task Force, pp. 39-47).

10. **(d)** The sensitivity and specificity of screening tests for prostate cancer cannot be determined with certainty. Biopsies are generally not performed on patients with negative screening test results, and this results in incomplete information about the number of true vs. false negative screenings. This makes it impossible to properly calculate sensitivity and specificity. Even digital rectal examinations, the oldest screening test for prostate cancer, have limited sensitivity and specificity because the examining finger can only palpate the posterior and lateral aspects of the gland; 25% to 35% tumors are inaccessible to the examining finger (USPS Task Force, pp. 19-29).

11. **(a)** Cancer of these structures is increased due to obesity and patients will benefit from knowing that there is a decrease in the incidence of these cancers as body weight is reduced (Rosenfeld, p. 83).

12. **(d)** The American Academy of Family Physicians recommends rubella antibody testing in all women of childbearing age who lack evidence of immunity. A tetanus booster and tuberculosis skin testing are important health maintenance and screening tests as well (USPS Task Force, pp. 278-279, 282-283, 361-368, 796-797).

13. **(b)** In settings where the prevalence of violence is high, clinicians should ask adolescents and young adults about previous violent behavior or victimization, current alcohol and drug use, and the availability of handguns and other firearms. There is currently insufficient evidence to recommend for or against clinician counseling to prevent morbidity and mortality with youth violence. Patients should be screened for problem drinking, signs and symptoms of drug abuse and dependence, the various presentations of family violence, and suicidal ideation in persons with established risk factors (USPS Task Force, pp. 687-693).

14. **(b)** Guidelines recommend a single pneumococcal vaccine for all healthy elderly over the age of 65, annual influenza vaccination starting at age 65 for healthy elderly clients, colorectal screening starting at age 50, and periodic cholesterol screening in low risk populations to begin at 35 to 65 for men and 45 to 65 for women. Earlier screening for cholesterol may be indicated based upon the recommendations of the National Heart, Lung, and Blood Institute's National Cholesterol Education Program. There is insufficient evidence to recommend for or against routine screening in children, adolescents, or low risk young adults (USPS Task Force, pp. 15, 89, 791).

References

Patem, R. R. (1995). Physical activity and public health: A recommendation from the Centers for Disease Control and Prevention and the American College of Sports Medicine. *Journal of the American Medical Association, 273*(5), 402-407.

Rosenfeld, J. (1997). *Women's health in primary care*. Baltimore: Williams & Wilkins.

U.S. Preventive Services (USPS) Task Force (1996). *Guide to clinical preventive services* (2nd ed.). Baltimore: Williams & Wilkins.

Dermatologic Disorders

Sharon Fruh

Select one best answer to the following questions.

A 26-year-old female day care worker, who is nursing a 4-month-old child, is complaining of intense itching at night. This started two days ago. On physical examination, the only significant finding is a rash in the interdigital areas and axilla. She has a positive burrow ink test.

1. Based on the above information, what is the best treatment choice for this patient?

    a. Permethrin 5%
    b. Lindane 1%
    c. Acyclovir
    d. Benzyl benzonate (25%)

Questions 2 and 3 refer to the following scenario.

A 25-year-old female presents with honey-colored crusts on her left forearm. A weeping erosion was noted when one of the honey crusts was gently moved. There is no surrounding erythema, and she has no lymphadenopathy. She states that her 4-year-old son was just treated for the same problem.

2. Based on the above information, what is the appropriate treatment for this patient?

    a. Triamcinolone 0.1% lotion
    b. Permethrin 5%
    c. Dicloxacillin
    d. Griseofulvin

3. Based on the above information, which of the following information would not be included in educating this patient?

a. Instruction for debridement of crust with wet soaks for 20 minutes t.i.d. followed by gentle scrubbing with a washcloth
b. That this condition is extremely contagious, and towels and washcloths used by the affected individual should be kept away from others
c. That fingernails should be kept short and scratching avoided
d. That treatment with topical agents is preferred over oral agents because they are equally effective

Questions 4 and 5 refer to the following scenario.

A 22-year-old female presents with a skin "problem" on her knees and elbows. According to the patient this started one month ago. She denies any change in her lifestyle or diet, and denies any family history of this problem. Physical examination reveals silvery looking scales and thickening on the extensor surfaces of both knees. The lesions have well demarcated borders and are symmetrical. The removal of a scale causes a small area of bleeding.

4. What is the first line of therapy based on the above information?

   a. Topical steroids
   b. Antibiotics
   c. Ultraviolet light
   d. Methotrexate

5. What underlying cause of this condition should be considered in individuals who have a sudden adult onset of this disease?

   a. Cancer
   b. Human immunodeficiency virus
   c. Diabetes
   d. Thyroid disorders

6. Which of the following treatments for psoriasis do not correspond with the side effects listed?

   a. PUVA—increased incidence of dermatologic malignancy
   b. Etretinate—teratogenicity
   c. High potency steroids—skin atrophy
   d. Anthralin—interferes with hair growth

Questions 7 and 8 refer to the following scenario.

A 33-year-old male presents with sores in his mouth which have been present for the last four days. He states that it really hurts to swallow. He denies similar symptoms in the past or recent change in diet. Physical examination of his mouth reveals white plaques on an erythematous base. Microscopically, a KOH preparation is positive. He states that he has had this condition before but that the last time it was also present in his esophagus.

7. Which of the following predisposing factors is least likely in this client?

    a. Use of inhaled steroids
    b. HIV positive status
    c. Diabetes mellitus
    d. Contact with an infected person

8. Based on the above information, what is the best treatment choice for this client?

    a. Nystatin
    b. Erythromycin
    c. Fluconazole
    d. Acyclovir

Questions 9, 10, and 11 refer to the following scenario.

An HIV positive patient reports itching and burning pain under his left arm extending to his back. He states that he had severe pain in that area a few days before the rash erupted. He also had a fever and a headache before the rash occurred. Physical examination reveals scattered confluent lesions with a dermatomal distribution line under the left axilla and extending to the posterior thorax. A skin scraping indicates a positive Tzanck smear.

9. Based on the above findings, what medication is most effective when started within 72 hours of the rash?

    a. Valacyclovir
    b. Ibuprofen
    c. Mupirocin
    d. Fluconazole

10. Which of the following topical therapies would not be recommended for application on the above patient's skin lesions?

   a. Burrow's solution
   b. Betadine solution
   c. Cool tap water compresses
   d. Salicylic preparations

This same patient returns to see you six days later and states that he never pur-chased his medication due to financial problems. He presents today because he now has this same rash above his left eye. He states that the pain is excruciating. Physi-cal examination reveals vesicular lesions that extend from around the left eye to the vertex of the skull.

11. Based on the above information, how would you alter your initial treatment plan?

   a. Refer him to an ophthalmologist for an extensive eye evaluation
   b. Start him on valacyclovir in the office and send him home with samples
   c. Refer him to a neurologist for an extensive evaluation
   d. Start him on fluconazole in the office and send him home with samples

12. Bill Lange is a 35-year-old client who complains of flu-like symptoms for the past four days. He states that he has not been exposed to anyone who has been sick; in fact, he just returned six days ago from a hunting trip in Wisconsin. Physical examination reveals a red ring lesion with partial central clearing on his left calf. Based on this information, what would be the drug treatment choice for this client?

   a. Amantadine
   b. Rimantadine
   c. Doxycycline
   d. Azithromycin

13. Which of the following would not be a potential long term consequence of un-treated Lyme disease?

   a. Episodes of arthritis
   b. Varying degrees of heart block
   c. Bell's palsy
   d. Cataracts

14. A 32-year-old male client presents with multiple scaly patches on his skin be-neath his beard. The Wood's light examination reveals green yellow fluores-cence of the hair shafts of his beard. The appropriate first line of treatment with this individual is:

a. Clotrimazole cream
b. Naftifine cream
c. Griseofulvin tablets
d. Selenium sulfide solution

15. A 26-year-old female presents with the complaint of intense itching of her scalp. Nits are identified upon examination of the hair shaft. What is the appropriate first line treatment for this condition?

a. Permethrin
b. Tretinoin
c. Trimethoprim/sulfamethoxazole
d. Benzoyl peroxide

16. Which of the following prescribing instructions for topical treatment of tinea versicolor is correct?

a. Clotrimazole—apply once daily for seven days, do not wash off
b. Ketoconazole—apply twice daily for seven days, do not wash off
c. Selenium sulfide suspension—apply once daily for seven days, wash off after 10 minutes
d. Lindane—apply once daily for seven days, wash off after 10 minutes

17. Which one of the following statements is false regarding the diagnosis of tinea versicolor?

a. A powdery scale can be demonstrated by scraping lightly with a #15 surgical blade
b. Hypha can be identified in a KOH treated scraping
c. Fluorescent areas can be identified using a Wood's light
d. White cells can be identified using a wet prep

18. A 17-year-old female with several small noninflamed acne lesions is best treated with:

a. Vibramycin
b. Isotretinoin
c. Tretinoin
d. Minocycline

19. Which of the following is not an appropriate guideline for the management of women being treated with isotretinoin?

    a. A baseline pregnancy test should be obtained, and contraception should be used while taking this medication and for one month afterward ⌐

    b. Vitamin supplements that contain vitamin A should not be used ⌐

    c. A patient taking this medication should not donate blood

    d. Triglyceride, CBC, and liver function tests should be done within two months of starting medication

Questions 20 and 21 refer to the following scenario.

Ms. Madison presents for evaluation of possible melanoma. She had a small melanoma lesion removed nine months ago and was advised to have her skin checked on a regular basis.

20. Which one of the following findings would not suggest that the new lesion is a melanoma?

    a. Asymmetry in the shape of the mole

    b. Border irregularity

    c. Color variation

    d. A 5 mm diameter

21. Ms. Madison's patient education includes teaching with regard to early diagnosis and treatment. Which of the following would not be an appropriate recommendation for this patient?

    a. Perform monthly self skin examinations

    b. Report any suspicious lesions at once

    c. Schedule follow-up visits every 12 months

    d. Avoid being in the sun at mid-day

22. Which of the following statements is false regarding the distribution of melanoma?

    a. The back is the most common site in males

    b. The legs are the most common site in females

    c. Melanoma can occur anywhere on the body

    d. Melanoma rarely occurs on the face

Answers and Rationale

1. **(a)** Permethrin 5%, a synthetic pyrethrin, is the drug of choice for treating scabies. It is safe and effective even in one treatment. It is safe for pregnant women and infants. Lindane should not be used in pregnancy or in nursing mothers, infants, or small children due to neurotoxicity (Rakel, pp. 992-993).

2. **(c)** This presentation is classic impetigo, a bacterial infection for which dicloxacillin is the drug of choice (Rakel, pp. 934-935).

3. **(d)** Options "a," "b," and "c" are all appropriate with regard to treating impetigo. However, topical antibiotics are not as effective as oral antibiotics in most settings (Tierney, et al., p. 141).

4. **(a)** Topical steroids are the appropriate first choice for treatment of psoriasis. Their potency increases when used under an occlusive dressing. Antibiotics are not effective unless there is an infection. Ultraviolet light is used with psoriasis, but not as a first line therapy. Methotrexate is reserved for severe cases after failure of other forms of therapy (Rakel, pp. 948-949).

5. **(b)** The sudden appearance of psoriasis may indicate a positive HIV status. One percent of HIV infected patients develop severe psoriasis that often presents as the initial symptom (Woolliscroft, p. 332).

6. **(d)** Anthralin can be applied once daily to the skin or scales but must be washed off within one hour because it can stain the skin. It does not interfere with hair growth (Rakel, pp. 948-949).

7. **(d)** Person to person spread generally does not occur with candida infections. Chronic or broad spectrum antibiotic use can be a predisposing factor as well as treatment with high dose corticosteriods, HIV, cancer chemotherapy, and hematological malignancy (Rakel, pp. 850-852).

8. **(c)** Fluconazole is the drug of choice. It is effective for oral and esophageal candidiasis. The nystatin oral suspension is effective for oral lesions but not as effective for esophageal lesions (Woolliscroft, p. 65; Rakel, p. 851).

9. **(a)** Antiviral therapy is the best treatment for acute herpes zoster in immuno-suppressed individuals (Woolliscroft, pp. 186-187).

10. **(d)** Topical salicylic preparations are used to treat the common wart. This would not be appropriate treatment for herpes zoster (Habif, pp. 352-359).

11. **(a)** It appears that he has ophthalmic zoster and should be referred to an ophthalmologist as a priority. Sight threatening complications can occur. Prompt treatment with acyclovir, administered intravenously to immuno-compromised patients, may reduce the severity of late ocular manifestations. (Habif, pp. 352-355).

12. **(c)** For adults in the early stages of illness from Lyme disease, doxycycline or amoxicillin is the treatment of choice. Amantadine and rimantadine are effective in treating individuals with influenza A (Habif, pp. 352-359; Dambro, p. 563).

13. **(d)** Of individuals with untreated Lyme disease, 60% develop arthritis, 8% develop heart problems such as AV block, and 15% exhibit nervous system involvement such as Bell's palsy (Habif, pp. 352-359; Dambro, p. 563).

14. **(c)** Single agent topical antifungals are ineffective in treating fungal infections of the scalp, beard area, or nails (Rakel, pp. 997-1000).

15. **(a)** Permethrin, a synthetic pyrethrin, is the most effective remedy available. It does not need to be repeated for head lice due to residual killing activity. It is available without a prescription. Lindane has been the standard therapy for many years, but reapplication in seven days is needed to kill hatching nits, and there is the risk of neurotoxicity when misused. Trimethoprim/sulfamethoxazole, one tablet twice daily for three days, is useful in severe infestations and needs to be repeated in 10 days (Rakel, pp. 997-1000; Habif, p. 456).

16. **(c)** Selenium sulfide suspension or shampoo needs to be applied once daily for seven days. Clotrimazole needs to be applied twice daily for several weeks. Ketoconazole should be applied once daily for one week. Lindane is used with lice treatment (Habif, p. 404; Dambro, pp. 1072-1073).

17. **(d)** A wet prep would identify trichomonas but not tinea versicolor (Habif, p. 404; Dambro, pp. 1072-1073, 1090).

18. **(c)** Small areas and superficial lesions should be treated with topical medication alone (Rakel, p. 932).

19. **(d)** Liver function tests, triglyceride, and complete blood counts need to be done prior to prescribing isotretinoin. Triglyceride levels are then performed at 2 to 3 weeks of treatment, then at four week intervals. CBC and liver function tests are performed at 4 to 6 weeks while on treatment (Habif, p. 166; Rakel, pp. 932-934).

20. **(d)** Diameter greater than 6 mm (about the size of a pencil eraser) is a key symptom that may indicate that a mole may be melanoma. However, these clinical warning signs do not apply to the nodular melanoma subtype (Rakel, pp. 932-934).

21. **(c)** This patient should be evaluated every six months after a personal history of early melanoma. Her relative risk of a second melanoma is increased 5 to 8 fold (Rakel, pp. 942-943).

22. **(d)** Melanoma can occur anywhere on the skin surface. However, it is more common to find melanoma in men on the area of the back, and women on the legs (Bergin, p. 780).

References

Bergin, J. D. (1997). *Medicine recall.* Baltimore: Williams & Wilkins.

Dambro, M. R. (1997). *Griffith's 5 minute clinical consult.* Baltimore: Williams & Wilkins.

Habif, T. (1996). *Clinical dermatology* (3rd ed.). St Louis: Mosby.

Rakel, R. E. (1996). *Saunders manual of medical practice.* Philadelphia: W. B. Saunders.

Tierney, Jr., L. M., McPhee, S. J., & Papadakis, M. A. (1998). *Current medical diagnosis and treatment* (37th ed.). Stamford, CT: Appleton & Lange.

Woolliscroft, J. O. (1997). *Handbook of current diagnosis and treatment.* St. Louis: Mosby.

Eye, Ear, Nose, and Throat Disorders

Sharon Fruh

Select one best answer to the following questions.

Questions 1 and 2 refer to the following scenario.

Mary Johnson presents with itching and burning in her left eye. She awoke this morning with her eyelashes matted shut. She states that her daughter recently had the same problem and was given some kind of drops. Physical examination of the eyes was significant for a slightly edematous left eyelid and injected left conjunctiva.

1. Based on the above information, what eye drops would not be appropriate for Mary?

    a. Sulfacetamide 10%
    b. Trimethoprim-polymyxin B
    c. Tobramycin 0.3%
    d. Trifluridine 1%

2. What advice would be appropriate for Mary in terms of general patient education?

    a. Use topical steroids if significant pain is present
    b. Use a patch on the left eye
    c. Use prescription drops in both eyes
    d. Use warm compresses to relieve discomfort

3. Mark, a 43-year-old patient, complains of frequent nasal congestion, nasal itching, and chronic clear postnasal drip. This started after his move to a warmer climate. Physical examination reveals pale, swollen turbinates. Nasal smears reveal eosinophils. Based on the above information, what medication would not be indicated?

    a. Loratadine
    b. Cromolyn sodium
    c. Azithromycin
    d. Beclomethasone

4. Jim, a 43-year-old patient, complains of a cold, low grade fever, mucopurulent nasal discharge, pain in his upper teeth, and facial pain when bending over. Physical examination is unremarkable except for tenderness over the maxillary sinuses. Based on the above information, what classification of medication would not be appropriate for Jim?

    a. Antibiotics
    b. Antihistamines
    c. Decongestants
    d. Mucolytics

5. Lynn, a 36-year-old patient, complains that upon awakening this morning there was a thick, yellow-green exudate "gumming" her lids. Physical examination reveals hyperemia and minimal itching. No preauricular adenopathy is noted. The Giemsa stain reveales neutrophils. Based on the above information, what classification of medication should be prescribed for Lynn?

    a. Antibiotic ointments
    b. Antiviral ointments
    c. Topical steroids
    d. Topical vasoconstrictors

6. You are concerned that Ms. Rachel has chronic sinusitis. Which of the following is not characteristic of chronic sinusitis?

    a. Symptoms that last beyond 21 days while on antibiotics
    b. Recurrence of symptoms in less than one month
    c. Three episodes in six months
    d. Two episodes in one year

7. Ms. Rachel has been treated for acute sinusitis. What additional organism(s) need(s) to be treated in chronic sinusitis?

    a. Staphylococci
    b. *H. influenzae*
    c. *Moraxella catarrhalis*
    d. Streptocci

8. Elizabeth is diagnosed with acute mononucleosis. Why would you avoid treating her with ampicillin?

    a. It is not effective against gram positive organisms
    b. It is not effective against gram negative organisms
    c. It can cause a maculopapular pruritic rash
    d. It can cause gastric ulcers

9. Hannah presents with hoarseness and dysphonia. She has an occasional nonproductive cough and complains of a slight sore throat. Physical examination is unremarkable. She is afebrile. Which of the following treatment modalities would not be appropriate at this point?

    a. Antibiotics
    b. Cough suppression
    c. Humidification
    d. Voice rest

10. Erik was diagnosed with a superficial corneal abrasion in his left eye. Which of the following would not be part of his initial treatment plan?

    a. Topical antibiotic drops
    b. Patching of the affected eye
    c. Contact lense removal
    d. Topical steroid drops

11. Aaron, a 40-year-old patient, has severe right otitis media. A Weber test would be expected to demonstrate:

    a. Sound equal in both ears
    b. Sound louder in the right ear
    c. Sound louder in the left ear
    d. Air conduction to bone conduction ratio 2:1 in both ears

12. In individuals who have had corneal foreign bodies removed, which ophthalmic medication should be avoided?

    a. Antibiotic ointment
    b. Saline drops
    c. Steroid drops
    d. Topical cycloplegics

13. Which of the following medications is the most effective treatment for uncomplicated influenza?

    a. Amantadine
    b. Acyclovir
    c. Cefaclor
    d. Itraconazole

14. Mr. Naman presents with a chronic elevation of intraocular pressure. Physical examination reveals visual field loss. He also has a positive history of asthma. Which of the following medications would be appropriate for his condition?

    a. Timolol
    b. Betaxolol
    c. Carteolol
    d. Trusopt

15. How often would you recommend Mr. Naman return for life long follow-up of his condition?

    a. Every two years
    b. Every 1 to 3 months
    c. Every nine months
    d. Every 4 to 6 months

Questions 16, 17, and 18 refer to the following scenario.

Mrs. Davis, a new patient, presents with a recent onset of a headache, left eye pain, blurred vision, and halos around lights. She is complaining of nausea. The only medications that she takes are an antihistamine and an antidepressant (she doesn't know the names). Physical examination reveals an intraocular pressure in her left eye of 73 mm Hg. Bilateral corneas are clear to inspection. The left lid is edematous with a fixed mid-dilated pupil noted.

16. These findings are consistent with which type of glaucoma?

    a. Infantile
    b. Borderline
    c. Chronic open-angle
    d. Primary angle-closure

17. What would be your treatment choice for Mrs. Davis?

    a. Prednisolone acetate
    b. Referral for hospital admission

   c. Acetazolamide

   d. Referral to an optometrist

18. What medication would not exacerbate Mrs. Davis' medical condition?

   a. Antihistamines

   b. Antidepressants

   c. Phenothiazines

   d. Beta blockers

19. Ms. Reed, a 30-year-old patient, presents today with an acute onset of dizziness. She states that she just recovered from an upper respiratory infection. Upon getting out of bed this morning, she became extremely dizzy. She states that if she lies very still she does not feel dizzy. When she sits up or stands, the dizziness returns. Physical examination reveals a positive paroxysmal positional vertigo. Based on this information and the most probable diagnosis, which of the following medications would not be appropriate?

   a. Dimenhydrinate

   b. Meclizine

   c. Promethazine

   d. Hydrochlorothiazide

20. Mr. Blake was recently diagnosed with recurring Meniere's disease. The maintenance management plan would not include:

   a. Bedrest during attacks

   b. Low salt diet

   c. Meclizine

   d. Aspirin

Answers and Rationale

1. **(d)** This condition appears to be a mild bacterial conjunctivitis which usually resolves in 1 to 3 days when treated with broad spectrum topical antibiotics. Answers "a," "b," and "c" are topical antibiotics which would be effective. Answer "d" is a topical antiviral medication which would be appropriate when the client has a viral conjunctivitis (Fihn & DeWitt, pp. 135-137; Dambro, pp. 254-255).

2. **(d)** Warm compresses are helpful if infective; cold compresses are helpful if allergic or irritative. Topical steroids are contraindicated in infectious conjunctivitis. Patching the left eye is not recommended. Using antibiotic drops in the unaffected eye is not recommended; it would only be appropriate to do this if the right eye became infected (Fihn & DeWitt, pp. 135-137; Dambro, pp. 254-255).

3. **(c)** In allergic rhinitis, antihistamines, cromolyn sodium, and topical steroids are all appropriate. Antibiotics are not indicated for this condition (Rakel, 1998, p. 768).

4. **(b)** These signs and symptoms are consistent with acute sinusitus. Decongestants and mucolytics are appropriate for symptom relief, and antibiotics are required. However, antihistamines may thicken nasal secretions and are not routinely indicated in the initial treatment of acute sinusitis (Rakel, 1996, pp. 90-92).

5. **(a)** A Giemsa stain that reveals neutrophils represents a bacterial infection. Mononuclear cells would have suggested a viral infection, and eosinophils would represent an allergic conjunctivitis (Rakel, 1996, pp. 69-71).

6. **(d)** More than four episodes per year is characteristic of chronic sinusitis (Bergin, p. 599).

7. **(a)** The same organisms that cause acute sinusitis may cause chronic sinusitis, as well as staphylococci and anaerobes (Bergin, p. 599).

8. **(c)** Ampicillin, when given to individuals who have the Epstein-Barr virus, has a 90% to 100% chance of provoking a maculopapular pruritic rash. Ampicillin is effective against gram negative and gram positive organisms. It is also a relatively inexpensive medication (Bergin, p. 462).

9. **(a)** Antibiotics are used only in selected patients when fever, productive cough, or purulent sputum are present. Otherwise voice rest, elimination of throat clearing, cough suppression, and humidification are the treatments for laryngitis (Rakel, 1996, pp. 108-109).

10. **(d)** Topical steroids are contraindicated because they retard healing and increase the risk of infection (Tierney, et al., p. 205).

11. **(b)** In conductive loss (such as with a severe otitis media), you would expect the sound to be louder in the affected ear. Normally the sound should be equal in both ears (Rakel, 1996, pp. 42-43).

12. **(c)** The use of steroids should be avoided because they may slow healing and can be dangerous in the circumstance of infection (Rakel, 1996, pp. 74-75).

13. **(a)** Amantadine is indicated for prophylaxis and treatment of influenza type A. Acyclovir is indicated for herpes zoster, chicken pox, and CMV. Cefaclor is a cephalosporin antibiotic. Itraconazole is an antifungal (Bergin, pp. 465-467; Ellsworth, et al., pp. 10-11, 23, 132-133, 446-447).

14. **(d)** Mr. Naman has chronic open angle glaucoma. Beta-adrenergic blocking agents are contraindicated with asthma (timolol, betaxolol, carteolol). Carbonic anhydrase inhibitors are not contraindicated with asthma (Fihn & DeWitt, pp. 130-132).

15. **(d)** Multiple visits are required to adjust therapy for individuals with chronic open angle glaucoma. Once stable, Mr. Naman needs to be monitored at least 2 to 4 times per year. Chronic carbonic anhydrase inhibitor therapy requires periodic monitoring of the blood count (hemoglobin, hematocrit, WBC and electrolytes) (Fihn & DeWitt, pp. 130-132; Dambro, pp. 426-427).

16. **(d)** Mrs. Davis has primary angle closure (acute) glaucoma (Dambro, pp. 428-429).

17. **(b)** Mrs. Davis needs to be admitted to the hospital for IV administration of medication. Antiemetics may be necessary, and surgical measures may be needed (Dambro, pp. 428-429; Fihn & Dewitt, pp. 130-133).

18. **(d)** The medications in answer choices "a," "b," and "c" may cause or exacerbate glaucoma (angle closure) in high risk individuals (Dambro, pp. 428-429).

19. **(d)** When treating acute labyrinthitis, antihistamines, antiemetics, and anticholinergics are appropriate. Hydrochlorothiazide is not an appropriate medication for this condition (Tierney, et al., p. 226).

20. **(d)** Ototoxic medications (aspirin, kanamycin, quinine) should be avoided. The patient should be encouraged to quit smoking, reduce stress, and avoid significant noise exposure by wearing ear protectors when necessary (Dambro, pp. 658-659).

References

Bergin, J. D. (1997). *Medicine recall*. Baltimore: Williams & Wilkins.

Dambro, M. R. (1997). *Griffith's 5 minute clinical consult*. Baltimore: Williams & Wilkins.

Ellsworth, A. J., Dugdale, D. C., Wit, D. M., & Oliver, L. M. (1997). *1997 medical drug reference*. St. Louis: Mosby.

Fihn, S. D., & DeWitt, D. E. (1998). *Outpatient medicine* (2nd ed.). Philadelphia: W. B. Saunders.

Rakel, R. E. (1998). *Conn's current therapy*. Philadelphia: W. B. Saunders.

Rakel, R. E. (1996). *Saunders manual of medical practice*. Philadelphia: W. B. Saunders.

Tierney, Jr., L. M., McPhee, S. J., & Papadikis, M. A. (1998). *Current medical diagnosis and treatment* (37th ed.). Stamford, CT: Appleton & Lange.

Respiratory Disorders

Cheryl Ahern-Lehmann

Select one best answer to the following questions.

A 35-year-old nurse comes into your occupational health clinic for a pre-employment physical examination. She tells you that she was born in Britain and received the BCG immunization as a child, so she has never been PPD skin tested in the U.S. Her last chest radiograph was three years ago and it was negative. She denies any known exposures to or symptoms of tuberculosis since that radiograph.

1. What would you do initially to rule out tuberculosis in this nurse?

   a. Order a chest radiograph and do a PPD (5 TU)
   b. A TB skin test with (5 TU) PPD
   c. A TB skin test with (1 TU) PPD
   d. Nothing this year, as she doesn't need another screening radiograph for two years

Questions 2 and 3 refer to the following scenario.

Mr. Huong, a 36-year-old Vietnamese man presents for a pre-employment physical. He has been newly hired for a night janitorial position in a dry cleaning business. He tells you that his Vietnamese mother-in-law lives in his home and is currently being treated for active tuberculosis. He denies any personal symptoms of tuberculosis, has no chronic illness, and uses no drugs regularly. He was PPD skin tested and had a chest radiograph eight months ago, after his mother-in-law's disease was discovered; both tests were negative at that time.

2. You place a PPD 5 TU on his right forearm. When he returns in 48 to 72 hours to have his skin test read, what minimum size of induration would you read as positive in this man?

   a. 3 mm
   b. 5 mm

    c. 10 mm

    d. 15 mm

3. If Mr. Huong's PPD was now positive, and a follow-up chest radiograph was negative, which of the following interventions would be appropriate?

    a. Begin prophylactic treatment with isoniazid 300 mg q.d. for 6 to 9 months

    b. Begin daily treatment with isoniazid, rifampin, and pyrazinamide

    c. Begin prophylactic treatment with standard doses of rifampin for six months

    d. Begin no pharmacologic treatment now but monitor for symptom development

4. Which of the following findings on a chest radiograph would be typical of a patient with primary active tuberculosis?

    a. Patchy or interstitial infiltrates in the lower lobes

    b. Small homogenous infiltrates in the upper lobes

    c. Decreased peripheral vascular markings, bullous lesions

    d. Cavitation in posterior apical segments

5. Of the following disorders, wheezing is least likely to occur in:

    a. Heart failure

    b. Pulmonary embolism

    c. Pneumonia

    d. Chronic bronchitis

Questions 6 and 7 refer to the following scenario.

A homeless man in his mid-fifties walks into the community clinic where you work. He is worried about a "terrible cough" he has developed over the last month. The cough occurs periodically throughout the day, but is "worse in the morning" when he coughs up "thick, smelly globs of brownish stuff." He says it doesn't have blood in it. He isn't sure whether the cough wakes him at night, because "he often gets drunk, passes out, and wakes up after sleeping it off somewhere on the sidewalk or in the park." He tells you that he sometimes "feels like he has a fever," but denies chills or "sweats." He has been losing weight. He proudly tells you he has never smoked. You order a radiograph; the results show small infiltrates in the posterior segment of the right upper lobe, the superior segment of the right lower lobe, and the basal segments of both lobes.

6. The diagnosis is most likely:

   a. Sarcoidosis
   b. Tuberculosis
   c. Aspiration pneumonia
   d. Viral pneumonia

7. Which of the following medications would you give this homeless man to treat his condition?

   a. Amoxicillin
   b. Ceftriaxone
   c. Rifampin
   d. Trimethoprim/sulfamethoxazole

Questions 8 and 9 refer to the following scenario.

Mr. Carney, a 60-year-old man with a 40-pack-year smoking history, presents with increasing dyspnea on exertion. He tells you he has noticed increasing amounts of blood in the sputum he "brings up" with his morning "smoker's cough." He is hoarse off and on, and his appetite is decreased. He has lost 10 pounds over the last three months.

8. Of the following diseases, which do you think is the most likely diagnosis for Mr. Carney?

   a. Chronic bronchitis
   b. Heart failure
   c. Bronchogenic carcinoma
   d. Chronic obstructive pulmonary disease

9. The initial test you would order to confirm Mr. Carney's diagnosis would be:

   a. Pulmonary function tests
   b. Complete blood count
   c. Blood gases
   d. Chest radiograph

10. Which of the following physical findings would you expect to find in a patient with pneumonia?

    a. Decreased fremitus and hyperresonance to percussion
    b. Increased fremitus and dullness to percussion
    c. Increased fremitus and hyperresonance to percussion

    d. Decreased fremitus and dullness to percussion

11. In patients with sarcoidosis, indications for treatment with oral corticosteroids include which of the following?

    a. Iritis
    b. Skin rashes
    c. Lymphadenopathy
    d. Chest radiograph with abnormal findings

12. Which of the following clinical conditions is not an underlying cause of pulmonary hypertension?

    a. Hepatic cirrhosis
    b. Emphysema
    c. Right ventricular failure
    d. Pulmonary embolism

13. A 23-year-old female comes in to see you, accompanied by a co-worker. The patient describes experiencing a sudden, brief, sharp pain in her left chest about 30 minutes ago while working at her desk. She fainted, then awoke feeling short of breath. She is dyspneic, diaphoretic, tachypneic, and very frightened; she is certain that she is having a heart attack. She denies any hypertension, cardiac problems or significant family history for cardiac problems. She is obese (5'3", 200 lbs), has varicose veins, and is on oral contraceptives. Upon examination, you note tachycardia, wheezes, crackles in her left posterior lung fields, and accentuation of the pulmonary component of the second heart sound. The most likely diagnosis is:

    a. Myocardial infarction
    b. Panic attack
    c. Asthma attack
    d. Pulmonary embolism

14. A 42-year-old migrant farm worker comes to the clinic because he "cannot shake a cold and flu that began three weeks ago." His symptoms started with a "runny nose, fever, chills, and body aches, like any flu." He then developed a dry, hacking cough productive of yellow sputum in the mornings. He has "a catching" pain when he takes a deep breath, and pain and swelling in his knees and ankles. This morning he developed three painful, red "bumps" on his right anterior shin. He is concerned that he may have had a significant exposure to pesticides last month when picking strawberries in Arizona. With this presentation, you are most concerned that this patient has developed:

a. Tuberculosis
b. Bacterial pneumonia
c. Coccidioidomycosis
d. Histoplasmosis

15. Which of the following is recommended initial treatment for *Pneumocystis carinii pneumonia* (PCP) in an AIDS patient?

a. Erythromycin
b. Trimethoprim/sulfamethoxazole
c. Azithromycin
d. Clindamycin

16. Which of the following medications is the first line treatment (after smoking cessation) in a patient with COPD?

a. Terbutaline MDI 2 puffs every 4 to 6 hours
b. Theophylline sustained release tablets 10 mg/kg/day in 1 to 3 doses
c. Beclomethasone MDI 2 puffs b.i.d.
d. Ipratropium bromide MDI 2 puffs q.i.d.

17. The organisms that cause the majority of cases of community-acquired pneumonia are:

a. *Streptococcus pneumoniae, Haemophilus influenzae, Mycoplasma pneumoniae*
b. *Haemophilus influenzae, Moraxella catarrhalis, Staphylococcus aureus*
c. *Streptococcus pneumoniae, Legionella* species, *Staphylococcus aureus*
d. *Moraxella catarrhalis, Mycoplasma pneumoniae, Klebsiella pneumoniae*

18. A 52-year-old male construction worker comes in to see you because he finds himself increasingly short of breath. He tells you that he smokes cigarettes, one half pack daily, and installs insulation in new houses, both of which he has done for 30 years. Upon physical examination you note inspiratory crackles and clubbing. His chest film is positive for interstitial fibrosis, thickened pleura, enlarged hilar lymph nodes with "eggshell" calcifications, small rounded opacities in his upper lung zones, and calcified pleural plaques on his diaphragm and lateral chest walls. His pulmonary function tests (PFT) indicate that he has restrictive lung disease. Your presumptive diagnosis for this man's lung disease is:

a. Silicosis
b. Asbestosis

   c. Tuberculosis
   d. Chronic bronchitis

19. Which one of the following drugs can cause a pleural effusion?

   a. Propranolol
   b. Inhaled cromolyn
   c. Aerosolized pentamidine
   d. Methysergide

20. A tall, thin, 22-year-old African-American male walks into the clinic because he has had some vague left-sided chest discomfort and shortness of breath for three days. Otherwise, he ''feels fine.'' He first noted the pain after ''rough-housing'' with some friends. He smokes cigarettes, one pack daily, but is otherwise "healthy." Upon examination he has a mild tachycardia, decreased tactile fremitus, diminished breath sounds, and hyperresonance over the lower one-third of his left posterior lung fields. You suspect this patient has a left lower lobe:

   a. Tension pneumothorax
   b. Spontaneous pneumothorax
   c. Bacterial pneumonia
   d. Pleuritis

21. Mrs. Little, a 65-year-old woman, presents for a routine annual physical examination. She is thin and tired appearing. She is "a pack a day" cigarette smoker (for 40 years), has a mild cough productive of small amounts of clear, mucoid sputum, she admits to increasing dyspnea ''almost all the time now,'' and has been losing weight. Upon physical examination she has diminished breath sounds, hyperresonance throughout her lung fields, and hypertrophied accessory respiratory muscles. Her laboratory work shows a normal hematocrit. She has a normal ECG, and an increased total lung capacity. Your diagnosis of this woman's respiratory disease is:

   a. Chronic bronchitis
   b. Emphysema
   c. Fibrotic lung disease
   d. Bronchogenic carcinoma

22. Which of the following is not a classic risk factor for adult respiratory distress syndrome (ARDS)?

   a. Aspiration of gastric contents

    b. Sepsis syndrome
    c. Circulatory shock
    d. Atypical pneumonia

Questions 23, and 24, and 25 refer to the following scenario.

A 25-year-old male comes to the clinic because he "can't shake this flu." He is most bothered by an intermittent, "severe hacking" cough, producing only small amounts of yellow sputum. His temperature is 99.6° F, and there are diffuse fine rales on physical examination. His chest radiograph shows extensive patchy infiltrates, but no consolidation. His CBC with differential shows no significant leukocytosis. He is a non-smoker, has no significant medical illness history, is on no medication regularly, and has no known drug allergies.

23. The most likely diagnosis for this patient is:

    a. Mycoplasma pneumonia
    b. Acute bronchitis
    c. Bacterial pneumonia
    d. Legionnaire's disease

24. Which one of the following antibiotics is recommended as the first line treatment for this young man's illness?

    a. Erythromycin
    b. Trimethoprim/sulfamethoxazole
    c. Cefuroxime
    d. Amoxicillin

25. How long after beginning treatment would you expect this young man's radiograph abnormalities to resolve?

    a. 10 days
    b. 2 weeks
    c. 3 weeks
    d. 4 weeks

Answers and Rationale

1. **(a)** Since this nurse is here for a pre-employment physical, and she falls into a high risk group (health care worker) for TB screening, a chest radiograph would be done to rule out active TB, and an intermediate strength PPD would be placed. Prior history of immunization with BCG vaccine as a child is not a total contraindication to the use of PPD skin testing; BCG is believed to provide immunity only for a short time. It has become common practice to do one intermediate strength (5 TU) PPD skin test to check baseline PPD reactions in people who were BCG immunized; this helps to determine the efficacy of PPD skin testing them in the future. Prior BCG vaccination may produce false positive indurations, but these are generally less than 10 mm in diameter. (Goroll, et al., p. 221; McColloster & Neff, p. 1580; Tierney, et al., p. 271; USPS Task Force, p. 278).

2. **(b)** This man falls in a high risk group. He is a close contact (lives in the same household) of an individual with active tuberculosis (Goroll, et al., p. 220; McColloster & Neff, p. 1580; Tierney, et al., p. 271).

3. **(a)** If Mr. Huong's PPD converted from eight months ago, he is at a 5% to 10% increased risk of developing tuberculosis within two years. Even though he is 36-years-old, he would be given INH prophylaxis for 6 to 9 months, if he had PPD skin reactivity of 5 mm or more, because he falls in a high risk group (close exposure to active tuberculosis) (Goroll, et al., p. 220; McColloster & Neff, p. 1582; Tierney, et al., p. 273-274).

4. **(b)** Small homogenous infiltrates in upper lobes, hilar and paratracheal lymph node enlargement, segmental atelectasis, and sometimes pleural effusion may be present in chest radiographs of primary active tuberculosis. Cavitory disease (as in option "d") and pulmonary infiltrates are suggestive of postprimary or reactivation tuberculosis. Patchy or interstitial infiltrates in the lower lobes are more characteristic of mycoplasma pneumonia, and the loss of pulmonary markings and bullous lesions are commonly seen with COPD (Tierney, et al., p. 270; Wells, et al., pp. 511, 1034).

5. **(c)** Wheezing is least likely to occur in pneumonia. Heart failure, pulmonary embolism and chronic bronchitis all frequently have wheezing as a physical finding. Pneumonia is a lower respiratory disease, with less involvement of the upper airways than the other conditions listed (Goroll, et al., p. 285).

6. **(c)** Aspiration pneumonia. Alcoholics have both diminished immune responses and a tendency to aspirate gastric or oropharyngeal contents (as do other patients with altered sensorium or neuromuscular diseases). Common etiologic agents include pneumococcus, *S. pneumoniae, S. aureus, H. influenzae*, and *Klebsiella pneumoniae*. This pneumonia is often "indolent with cough, low grade fever and weight loss, although an acute presentation may occur. Rigors are notably absent, but putrid sputum can be suggestive of the diagnosis." Chest radiographs show infiltrates in dependent lung segments, a common finding in "the somnolent alcoholic" (Wells, et al., pp. 41-42; Stobo, et al., p. 129).

7. **(b)** Treatment recommendations for alcoholics with aspiration pneumonia include the use of a second or third generation cephalosporin or an aminoglycoside (Stobo, et al., p. 131; Wells, et al., p. 512).

8. **(c)** Dyspnea, cough with blood-tinged sputum, hemoptysis, hoarseness, anorexia, and weight loss (particularly in an older patient, who has a long-time smoking history), are symptoms of bronchogenic carcinoma (Goroll, et al., p. 295; Tierney, et al., p. 277).

9. **(d)** Patients with suspected lung cancer should receive a complete blood count, liver function tests, and measurement of serum electrolytes and calcium, in addition to a chest radiograph. While the blood gases and PFT may give the clinician a sense of his pulmonary status, they are not part of the initial evaluation for lung cancer. Later definitive diagnosis requires cytologic or histologic evidence of cancer (Tierney, et al., p. 277).

10. **(b)** One would expect to find increased fremitus and dullness to percussion over areas of lung consolidation (Tierney, et al., pp. 237-238).

11. **(a)** Iritis. Indications for treating a sarcoid patient with oral corticosteroids include signs of significant or progressive involvement of any organ, or persistent constitutional symptoms such as fever, fatigue, hypercalcemia, iritis, arthritis, hepatitis, myocardial conduction defects, facial nerve palsies, cutaneous or symptomatic pulmonary lesions. Skin rashes, lymphadenopathy, and asymptomatic chest radiograph changes are earlier signs of sarcoid which do not require treatment with corticosteroids (Goroll, et al., p. 281; Tierney, et al., p. 287).

12. **(c)** Right ventricular failure is a result of pulmonary hypertension, not a cause. Hepatic cirrhosis, emphysema, and pulmonary embolism can all cause or lead to pulmonary hypertension (Tierney, et al., p. 298).

13. **(d)** This patient's history and physical findings are clinically suggestive of pulmonary embolism, and she also has several risk factors for pulmonary embolism; obesity, varicosities, and estrogen in oral contraceptives (Tierney, et al, p. 293; Weinstock & Neides, p. 82).

14. **(c)** Coccidioidomycosis results from inhalation of *Coccidioides immitis*, a mold that grows in soil in certain arid regions of the southwestern U.S. A migrant farm worker who had been picking strawberries in Arizona would be at high risk for this disease. In addition, his influenza-type symptoms, knee and ankle symptoms, and erythema nodosum lesions are characteristic of the presentation of coccidioidomycosis (Tierney, et al., pp. 1358-1359).

15. **(b)** Trimethoprim/sulfamethoxazole is considered first line treatment for *Pneumocystis carinii* pneumonia in an AIDS patient (Tierney, et al., p. 1361; Weinstock & Neides, p. 248).

16. **(d)** Ipatropium bromide is the first line treatment (after smoking cessation) in a patient with COPD, because it is superior to other drugs in achieving bronchodilation in patients with COPD (Tierney, et al., p. 252; Weinstock & Neides, p. 119).

17. **(a)** *Streptococcus pneumoniae, Haemophilus influenzae*, and *Mycoplasma pneumoniae* are the organisms that currently cause the majority of cases of community acquired pneumonia in the United States (Cunha, et al., p. 145; Tierney, et al., pp. 261-262).

18. **(a)** The occupation, physical findings, radiologic and PFT changes listed in this case are consistent with a diagnosis of silicosis (Goroll, et al., pp. 224-225; Tierney, et al., pp. 303-304).

19. **(d)** Methysergide is one of many drugs that can cause physiologic changes that lead to the development of pleural effusions (Tierney, et al., pp. 305, 317).

20. **(b)** Spontaneous pneumothorax commonly occurs in tall, thin men and presents with pleuritic pain (often a vague unilateral chest discomfort) and dyspnea. Mild tachycardia, decreased tactile fremitus, diminished breath sounds, and hyperresonance over the involved lung fields are typical clinical findings (Goroll, et al., p. 95; Tierney, et al., pp. 317-318).

21. **(b)** The classic description of a patient with emphysema is age 50, thin and wasted in appearance, pursed lip breathing, and constant, progressive dyspnea worsened on exertion. There is often a mild to moderate cough productive of clear, mucoid sputum. Upon examination the emphysemic patient has an increased anteroposterior chest diameter, with hypertrophied accessory respiratory muscles, diminished breath sounds, and hyperresonance on percussion. Hematocrit and ECG are commonly normal/negative, and PFT shows increased total lung capacity (Goroll, et al., p. 252; Tierney, et al., p. 251).

22. **(d)** Atypical (mycoplasma) pneumonia is not a classic risk factor for the development of ARDS, as are the other choices listed as answer options in this question (Tierney, et al., pp. 311-312).

23. **(a)** This patient's symptoms and findings are consistent with a diagnosis of mycoplasma pneumonia (what used to be called atypical pneumonia). He is young, basically healthy, and "less sick" (no high fever or chills) than a patient with bacterial pneumonia. His cough is hacking in quality, not significantly productive, and he has had systemic "flu-like" symptoms (Cunha, et al., p. 158; Goroll, et al., pp. 288-289; Tierney, et al., pp. 261-263).

24. **(a)** Erythromycin is the first line antibiotic treatment recommended for *mycoplasma pneumoniae* (Stobo, et al., p. 131; Wells, et al., p. 512).

25. **(d)** Radiograph abnormalities resolve slowly with *Mycoplasma pneumoniae*; it may take 4 to 6 weeks for complete resolution (Wells, et al., p. 512).

References

Cunha, B. A., Segreti, J., & Yamauchi, T. (1996). Community-acquired pneumonia: New bugs, new drugs. *Patient Care, 30*(5), 142-162.

Goroll, A. H., May, L. A., & Mulley, A. G. (1995). *Primary care medicine* (3rd ed.). Philadelphia: J. B. Lippincott.

McColloster, P., & Neff, N. E. (1996). Outpatient management of tuberculosis. *American Family Physician, 53*(3), 1579-1586.

Stobo, J. D., Hellmann, D. B., Ladenson, P. W., Petty, B. G., & Traill, T. A. (Eds.). (1996). *The principles and practice of medicine* (23rd ed.). Stamford, CT: Appleton & Lange.

Tierney, Jr., L. M., McPhee, S. J., & Papadakis, M. A. (1998). *Current medical diagnosis and treatment* (37th ed.). Stamford, CT: Appleton & Lange.

U.S. Preventive Services (USPS) Task Force. (1996). *Guide to clinical preventive services* (2nd ed.). Baltimore: Williams & Wilkins.

Weinstock, M. B., & Neides, D. M. (1996). *The resident's guide to ambulatory care* (2nd ed.). Columbus, OH: Anadem Publishing.

Wells, B. G., DiPiro, J. T., Schwinghammer, T. L., & Hamilton, C. W. (1998). *Pharmacotherapy handbook.* Stamford, CT: Appleton & Lange.

Cardiovascular Disorders

Sharon Fruh

Select one best answer to the following questions.

Questions 1 and 2 refer to the following scenario.

1. Mr. Baker, a 57-year-old patient with type 2 diabetes, is diagnosed with primary hypertension. Which class of antihypertensive medication should be avoided in this patient?

    a. ACE inhibitor
    b. Beta blocker
    c. Calcium channel blocker
    d. Alpha blocker

2. Mr. Baker also has proteinuria. Which antihypertensive medication would be the best choice for him?

    a. ACE inhibitor
    b. Beta blocker
    c. Calcium channel blocker
    d. Thiazide diuretics

3. Mr. Timothy, a 62-year-old male who is being treating for hypertension, complains of a very aggravating, intermittent cough. This cough started shortly after he started a new antihypertensive medication. Mr Timothy is most likely taking which type of medication?

    a. ACE inhibitor
    b. Beta blocker
    c. Calcium channel blocker
    d. Thiazide diuretics

4. Mrs. Hannah, a 72-year-old female client who has hypertension, is being treated with a diuretic. She reports that she has been taking nonsteroidal anti-

inflammatory medications daily the last two weeks for her arthritis. This is a concern since it is known that these medications affect the antihypertensive action of diuretics by:

    a. Enhancing the efficacy
    b. Blunting the effects
    c. Prolonging the action
    d. Potentiating the response

5. Mr. Richards has had three separate blood pressure readings of greater than 160/100 mm Hg. He is presently being treated for gout. Which antihypertensive medication would not be appropriate for him?

    a. Diuretic
    b. Beta blocker
    c. Calcium channel blocker
    d. Alpha blocker

6. Which of the following statements is not true with regard to the treatment of hypertension and the progression of treatment with first line agents?

    a. If hypertension is not initially controlled on a first line medication, the dose should be maximized
    b. If hypertension is not controlled with maximal doses of a first line agent, another first line agent should be added
    c. In asymptomatic patients, allow 2 to 4 weeks between dose or medication changes
    d. The goal of therapy is to reduce blood pressure below 120/80 mm Hg

7. Susan, a 62-year-old, recently had a myocardial infarction with resultant left ventricular systolic dysfunction. What antihypertensive medication would be the most beneficial in light of her cardiac condition?

    a. ACE inhibitor
    b. Thiazide diuretic
    c. Calcium channel blocker
    d. Alpha blocker

8. Which of the following instructions is not appropriate when teaching a client to manage infrequent attacks of stable angina?

    a. Instruct the client to sit down before taking nitroglycerin
    b. Advise the client to wait five minutes before taking another nitroglycerin tablet

    c. Advise the client to call 911 if pain is not relieved after three tablets or if tablets must be taken more often than every 30 to 60 minutes

    d. Remind the client that nitroglycerin should only be used when the pain is unbearable

9. A 58-year-old hypertensive male is diagnosed with arterial insufficiency of the extremities. He has smoked two packs of cigarettes per day for the past 30 years and is 30 pounds over his ideal body weight. He describes a cramping pain in both calves when he walks for more than 10 minutes. He also states that he has become impotent over the past six months. Management of this condition is multifaceted. As part of this treatment plan, this patient would not be advised to:

    a. Refrain from tobacco products

    b. Lose weight

    c. Walk daily to the point of discomfort

    d. Wear loose fitting shoes

10. J. Ryan, a 49-year-old male, presents with left calf pain and localized swelling and tenderness. He was discharged from the hospital two days ago following arthroscopic surgery to his left knee. He states that he has not been on any medication since his surgery. On physical examination the left calf is warm, swollen, and painful to palpation. He has a positive Homan's sign and a low grade temperature. What is the first step in the treatment plan of this patient?

    a. Physician referral

    b. Heparin therapy

    c. Ampicillin

    d. Coumadin therapy

11. A healthy, 38-year-old male suddenly develops atrial fibrillation. A thorough history is obtained to elicit any possible precipitating causes. Which of the following initial diagnostic tests is not necessary?

    a. 12 lead electrocardiogram

    b. Thyroid function tests

    c. Electrolytes, BUN and creatinine

    d. Hepatitis profile

12. When a patient presents with atrial fibrillation, what serious consequence can result from this condition?

    a. Sick sinus syndrome

b. Cerebrovascular accident
c. Mitral valve disease
d. Tricuspid valve disease

13. In individuals with persistent atrial fibrillation, which class of medication should be considered for rate control before elective cardioversion is considered?

a. Diuretics
b. Digitalis glycosides
c. Antibiotics
d. Anticoagulants

14. Which of the following uncomplicated, noncardiac causes of chest pain requires a physician consultation?

a. Herpes zoster
b. Respiratory infections
c. Mild gastrointestinal problems
d. Rib fractures

15. Ms. Jones presents here for a follow-up appointment following an acute myocardial infarction two months ago. Which one of the following medications should not be in her current treatment plan?

a. Aspirin
b. Streptokinase
c. Beta blocker
d. ACE inhibitor

Questions 16, 17, and 18 refer to the following scenario.

A 36-year-old female complains of chest pain aggravated by coughing, twisting, and deep inspiration. She has had a chest cold for three weeks and has coughed excessively. Physical examination identifies tenderness to rib palpation bilaterally, especially on the left side. Lungs are clear to auscultation.

16. What is the appropriate class of medications to prescribe for this patient based on the above information?

a. NSAID
b. Corticosteriod

    c. Cough suppressant
    d. Macrolides

17. This individual should be instructed to:

    a. Rest in bed for at least 72 hours to decrease the chance of complications
    b. Apply cold compresses to the area for twenty minutes three times a day
    c. Refrain from excessive use or aggravation of the pectoralis major muscle
    d. Avoid stretching exercises for at least three weeks after improvement of symptoms

18. When assessing and treating individuals with this condition, what important principle should the NP always remember?

    a. It tends to improve quickly and rarely recurs
    b. It may coexist with other diseases
    c. It occurs more commonly in men
    d. It occurs most commonly in the 5th to 6th decade of life

Questions 19 and 20 refer to the following scenario.

A 72-year-old obese male complains of the following symptoms that have progressed over the past two years: Dyspnea on exertion, fatigue, swollen ankles, and shortness of breath at night. On physical examination you identify jugular venous distention at 45 degrees, tachycardia, hypotension, an S_3 heart sound, pulmonary rales, edema, and hepatomegaly. Chest radiograph indicates left ventricular hypertrophy, and ECG demonstrates conduction abnormalities.

19. This patient's signs, symptons and diagnostic findings are most consistent with:

    a. Tricuspid valve disease
    b. Mitral valve disease
    c. Aortic valve disease
    d. Congestive heart failure

20. When treating the above patient with a stepwise approach, what classification of medication would you ideally prescribe for your patient in addition to a diuretic?

    a. ACE inhibitor
    b. Calcium channel blocker

   c. Beta blocker

   d. Antiarrhythmic agent

Questions 21 and 22 refer to the following scenario.

Ms. Roth, a 29-year-old female, has come in for an employment physical. Her history is unremarkable. Physical examination of her heart identifies a mid systolic click and a late systolic regurgitation murmur.

21. Which test is most appropriate to confirm the suspected diagnosis?

   a. Echocardiography

   b. Exercise stress test

   c. Cardiac catherization

   d. CT scan

22. What is the treatment choice for this patient?

   a. Valve replacement

   b. Antibiotic prophylaxis

   c. Loop diuretics

   d. ACE inhibitors

23. Which of the following statements is true with regard to treating aortic stenosis?

   a. Anticoagulants are often recommended

   b. The most effective treatment is ACE inhibitors

   c. Vasodilators can cause irreversible hypotension

   d. Pacemakers can be beneficial

24. A 30-year-old female presents with classic symptoms of Raynaud's syndrome. She lives in a cold climate and seems to need medication during the winter months. Which medication would not be appropriate for her?

   a. Nifedipine

   b. Diltiazem

   c. Prazosin

   d. Quinaglute

Answers and Rationale

1. **(b)** Beta-blocker use in patients with diabetes can mask symptoms produced by counter regulatory hormones and delay the systemic response to hypoglycemia (JNC VI, p. 2438).

2. **(a)** ACE inhibitors retard the progression of diabetic nephropathy (JNC VI, p. 2438).

3. **(a)** ACE inhibitors tend to produce a chronic, dry cough in about 15% of patients (Tierney, et al., p. 442; Noble, p. 193).

4. **(b)** NSAID may produce sodium retention and blunt the antihypertensive effect of diuretics (Noble, p. 195).

5. **(a)** All diuretics can increase serum uric acid levels in patients with gout (JNC VI, p. 2439).

6. **(d)** The goal of therapy is to reduce pressures below 140/90 mm Hg without adverse effects (Tierney, et al., p. 435).

7. **(a)** ACE inhibitors are useful after MI to prevent subsequent heart failure and mortality according to the sixth report of the JNC (JNC VI, p. 2439).

8. **(d)** Always incorporate into the teaching plan that nitroglycerin is used for chest pain at the onset of pain. Pain that persists or is not relieved in a patient with known or suspected heart disease requires immediate evaluation. Repeated use is not harmful or addictive (Rakel, 1996, p. 221).

9. **(d)** Avoid injury to the feet by wearing well fitting shoes. Shoes should not be loose but should fit properly. It is also best to avoid extremes of temperature of the feet. It is well documented that a training program of walking can reduce the onset of claudication symptoms, enhance resting blood flow, and increase maximal walking time. The use of vasodilating drugs has not been beneficial to all individuals with this problem, and literature does not support generalized use. Indications for operation include ischemic pain or tissue loss (Rakel, 1996, pp. 209-211).

10. **(a)** Referral or consultation is indicated for this patient. Orthopedic surgery is a major risk factor for DVT (Rakel, 1996, pp. 283-285).

11. **(d)** A 12 lead ECG is essential. Thyroid function tests are necessary to rule out hyperthyroidism as the cause of the atrial fibrillation. Electrolytes, BUN, and creatinine are indicated. A hepatitis profile is not necessary. (Dambro, pp. 104-105).

12. **(b)** A real concern in the management of patients with atrial fibrillation is the risk of cerebrovascular accident. The fibrillating atria provide an opportunity for thrombus formation, which could detach and travel to the brain or other critical areas of the body. Individuals with intermittent atrial fibrillation are at greater risk when they resume sinus rhythm, as clots may dislodge when a normal rhythm is re-established (Rakel, 1996, p. 273; Fihn & DeWitt, p. 255-261).

13. **(b)** Three main categories of drugs are used to block the atrioventricular (AV) node in an attempt to slow the ventricular response in atrial fibrillation; digitalis glycosides, beta-adrenergic blockers, and calcium channel blockers (Rakel, 1998, p. 262; Fihn & DeWitt, pp. 255-261).

14. **(d)** Rib fractures often accompany chest trauma, and the nurse practitioner should consult with or refer to a physician. With rib fractures, one must always rule out cardiac contusion, traumatic pericarditis, laceration of the great vessels, ruptured spleen, hepatic contusion, pneumothorax or hemothorax, and pulmonary contusion (Rakel, 1996, pp. 168-169).

15. **(b)** Streptokinase is a thrombolytic agent that is used immediately following onset of an MI to lyse the thrombosis. At one month post MI, most clients are on either aspirin or coumadin. Most patients are put on beta blockers after an MI for at least two years. ACE inhibitors are also being used and result in fewer recurrent ischemic events and less ventricular enlargement (Rakel, 1996, pp. 231-234).

16. **(a)** A nonsteroidal anti-inflammatory medication is the treatment of choice for costochondritis. Analgesics or salicylates are also often used. Corticosteroid

injection is sometimes indicated for patients refractory to usual measures. Local heat is also used as adjunct therapy. Cough suppressants are rarely indicated for any condition. Macrolides are indicated for management of pneumonia, but there is no clear evidence that this patient has pneumonia (Rakel, 1996, pp. 785-786; Dambro, pp. 264-265).

17. **(c)** Bedrest is not necessary with costochondritis. Instead of cold compresses, local heat should be applied. Advise her to refrain from movements that would aggravate the pectoralis major muscle. It is important to participate in stretching exercises (not overuse) for at least three weeks after the improvement of symptoms (Rakel, 1996, pp. 785-786; Dambro, p. 264-265).

18. **(b)** This condition improves over time but often recurs. Costochondritis occurs more commonly in women in the 20 to 40 age range. This condition may coexist with other disease processes such as atherosclerotic disease, so it is important that other disease processes be ruled out and not overlooked (Rakel, 1996, pp. 785-786; Dambro, pp. 264-265).

19. **(d)** Based on the history, physical, and diagnostic tests, this patient clearly suffers from congestive heart failure. The symptoms suggest both right and left ventricular failure. Left ventricular failure is the most common type with symptoms of pulmonary congestion. Right ventricular failure has features of systemic congestion (Rakel, 1998, pp. 292-294; Tierney, et al., p. 405).

20. **(a)** ACE inhibitors have become standard therapy for heart failure. They are helpful because they cause vasodilation and inhibit increased neurohormonal activity. Although beta blockers prolong survival in ischemic disease they may worsen heart failure (Rakel, 1998, pp. 294-296; Tierney, et al., pp. 407-411).

21. **(a)** Echocardiography is used to confirm the diagnosis (Dambro, pp. 684-685; Rakel, 1996, pp. 257-258).

22. **(b)** In asymptomatic individuals with an audible murmur, the necessary treatment is antibiotic prophylaxis for dental and surgical procedures. If this disease progresses, then she may be a candidate for diuretics and anticoagulation (Dambro, pp. 684-685; Rakel, 1996, pp. 256-258).

23. **(c)** Vasodilators in aortic stenosis are very dangerous. They can cause irreversible hypotension (Rakel, 1996, p. 259).

24. **(d)** Quinaglute is an antidysrhythmic medication and is not appropriate for Raynaud's disease. The most effective medication with Raynaud's disease is nifedipine. The use of diltiazem, verapamil, reserpine, methyldopa, and prazosin have equivocal support in the literature. 90% of patients respond favorably to smoking cessation, discontinuing offending medications, limiting occupational exposure to offending vibratory tools, and wearing mittens in cold weather (Dambro, pp. 898-899).

References

Dambro, M. R. (1997). *Griffith's 5 minute clinical consult*. Baltimore: Williams & Wilkins.

Fihn, S. D., & DeWitt, D. E. (1998). *Outpatient medicine* (2nd ed.). Philadelphia: W. B. Saunders.

Noble, J. (Ed.). (1996). *Textbook of primary care medicine*. (2nd ed.). (St Louis: Mosby.

Rakel, R. E. (1998). *Conn's current therapy*. Philadelphia: W. B. Saunders..

Rakel, R. E. (1996). *Saunders manual of medical practice*. Philadelphia: W. B. Saunders.

The sixth report of the joint national committee on detection, education, and treatment of high blood pressure (JNC VI). (1997). *Archives of Internal Medicine. 157,* 2413-2439.

Tierney, Jr., L. M., McPhee, S. J., & Papadakis, M. A. (1998). *Current medical diagnosis and treatment* (37th ed.). Stamford, CT: Appleton & Lange.

Hematology/Oncology Disorders

Cheryl Ahern-Lehmann

Select one best answer to the following questions.

1. The NP draws a screening CBC during a routine annual examination of a 50-year-old male. There are no significant health problems in his history. The results are as follows: Hemoglobin, 12 g/dL; hematocrit, 36%; MCV, 104 μ^3. Based upon these test results, this patient may have which of the following conditions?

    a. Iron deficiency anemia
    b. Anemia of chronic disease
    c. Folate deficiency anemia
    d. Aplastic anemia

Questions 2 and 3 refer to the following scenario.

68-year-old Margaret Green presents for a screening physical examination. She reports no chronic health problems and takes no medications regularly. She says that she has been experiencing some fatigue, "dizziness and balance problems," "trouble with memory," and "a little depression" over the last two months. The rest of the review of systems is negative, except for a "sore tongue." Her screening CBC suggests an anemia, with a hematocrit of 25%, and a hemoglobin of 10 g/dL. You order follow-up blood tests and get the following results: Serum iron, 50 μg/dL; serum folic acid, 6 ng/mL; serum vitamin B_{12}, 90 pg/mL. The laboratory also did a peripheral blood smear and found hypersegmented neutrophils.

2. Given these test results, which of the following tests would you order next to help you determine the underlying cause of Mrs. Green's anemia?

    a. Serum ferritin
    b. Red blood cell folate level
    c. Direct Coombs test
    d. Schilling test

3. Based on Mrs. Green's test results, which of the following treatments would you most likely recommend for her?

   a. Ferrous sulfate
   b. Vitamin B_{12} injections
   c. Folate
   d. Multivitamin

4. A 25-year-old woman suffers acute blood loss after a motor vehicle accident. Her CBC will most likely demonstrate an MCV in which of the following ranges?

   a. 40 to 60 μ^3
   b. 60 to 80 μ^3
   c. 80 to 100 μ^3
   d. 100 to 120 μ^3

5. The most common cause of iron deficiency anemia in a 38-year-old adult male would be?

   a. Alcoholism
   b. Gastrointestinal blood loss
   c. Chronic inflammatory bowel disease
   d. Malnutrition

6. The differential diagnosis for iron deficiency anemia includes which of the following?

   a. Thalassemia
   b. Folate deficiency
   c. Aplastic anemia
   d. Vitamin B_{12} deficiency

7. The NP performs a routine screening examination on Ms. Leong, a healthy 22-year-old Vietnamese woman. Her laboratory studies indicate that she has a microcytic, hypochromic anemia. In a follow-up visit you discuss this finding with her. Her history is negative for symptoms and known causes of anemia. You then order more tests to rule out iron deficiency, and all of those tests come back suggesting that iron deficiency is not the source of her anemia. You begin to consider that the cause for Ms. Leong's microcytic anemia could be thalassemia. Which of the following hematology tests would you order to determine if thalassemia is the underlying cause?

    a. Plasma erythropoietin level and blood smear for morphology
    b. Red cell distribution width (RDW) and bone marrow aspirate
    c. Hemoglobin electrophoresis and plasma erythropoietin level
    d. Hemoglobin electrophoresis and blood smear for morphology

8. It is recommended that women take folate supplementation during pregnancy, in order to:

    a. Prevent folate deficiency anemia
    b. Reduce cardiac risk of the mother
    c. Prevent cardiac abnormalities in the fetus
    d. Reduce the risk of neural tube defects in the fetus

9. Which of the following is a possible cause of megaloblastic anemia?

    a. Lead toxicity
    b. Sickle cell abnormalities
    c. Chemotherapy
    d. Renal failure

10. Which of the following WBC (white blood cell) counts represents a "shift to the left" suggesting bacterial infection?

    a. WBC 7,000 mm^3; neutrophils 50%; 2-3% segs/bands
    b. WBC 10,000 mm^3; neutrophils 35%; 8-10% segs/bands
    c. WBC 13,000 mm^3; neutrophils 85%; 15-17% segs/bands
    d. WBC 16,000 mm^3; neutrophils 10%; 10-12% segs/bands

11. Mrs. Jones, a 30-year-old woman, comes into your office because she is concerned about her increasing fatigue. When questioned she tells you that she is three months pregnant, finds herself increasingly out of breath when she goes up stairs, and has a frequent desire to suck on ice. These symptoms might all be due to her pregnancy, but you want to be certain that she is not anemic. Given the presentation and symptoms, which of the following anemias is most likely?

    a. Folate deficiency anemia
    b. Iron deficiency anemia
    c. Pernicious anemia
    d. Aplastic anemia

12. When evaluating the therapeutic efficacy of your treatment of a patient with

iron deficiency anemia, when would you expect to see the reticulocyte count increase?

   a. 7 to 10 days
   b. 3 weeks
   c. 1 month
   d. 3 months

13. Severe dysplasia (carcinoma in situ) is considered class IV (high grade squamous intraepithelial lesions [HGSIL]) in the Bethesda system of classifying Pap smears. It is considered what level of pathology in the CIN classification system?

   a. CIN I
   b. CIN II
   c. CIN III
   d. CIN IV

14. Which of the following is not considered a risk factor for breast cancer?

   a. Early age of menarche
   b. Biological father with history of breast cancer
   c. Maternal aunt with history of breast cancer
   d. Early age of first live birth

15. Teaching men to examine their own testicles in order to identify early signs of testicular cancer is most critical in which of the following age groups?

   a. Ages 13 to 19 years
   b. Ages 20 to 39 years
   c. Ages 40 to 59 years
   d. Ages 60 to 79 years

16. Which of the following individuals is at greatest risk of developing cervical cancer?

   a. An African-American woman who has multiple sexual partners
   b. A Caucasian woman who has multiple sexual partners
   c. A teenager who uses oral contraceptives
   d. A menopausal woman on hormone replacement therapy

17. Ten to 20% of cancer patients will develop hypercalcemia at some point during the course of their illness. Patients with which of the listed cancers are least likely to develop hypercalcemia?

    a. Colon cancer
    b. Lung cancer
    c. Multiple myeloma
    d. Breast cancer

18. A 39-year-old female nurse working with you in the clinic suddenly finds herself unable to speak clearly, or to use her dominant right hand. Her symptoms remain unchanged for over 48 hours, and her initial evaluation documents a stroke of uncertain etiology. She takes no medications regularly, and has no significant physical, historical, or family risk factors for heart disease or stroke. Her treating clinicians begin to believe that she has experienced a hypercoagulatory episode, and begin an evaluation to determine the source of her stroke. Which of the following diseases would not be considered in their differential diagnosis, since it is not a cause of hypercoagulatory states?

    a. Uremia
    b. Pregnancy
    c. Cancer
    d. Ulcerative colitis

19. Which of the following drugs is known to increase the prothrombin time (PT) and international normalized ratio (INR) when used in conjunction with coumadin?

    a. Penicillin
    b. Hydrochlorthiazide
    c. Trimethoprim/sulfamethoxazole
    d. Acetaminophen

20. Which of these statements is not correct with regard to current recommendations for the management of cancer pain?

    a. Meperidine is the preferred and most commonly recommended opioid analgesic for treatment of long term cancer pain
    b. The need for increasing doses of opioid analgesic, the development of opioid tolerance, and physical dependence often reflects the progression of the cancer
    c. Clinicians should not withhold increasingly high doses of opioid needed for pain relief, even when there is risk of side effects
    d. Patients receiving opioid analgesics "by the clock" should be provided additional oral or parenteral rapid onset, short duration opioids for breakthrough pain, as needed

Answers and Rationale

1. **(c)** A MCV of 104 μ^3 is indicative of a macrocytic anemia. The only macrocytic anemia on the list is folate deficiency anemia (Goroll, p. 449; Tierney, et al., p. 480; Wells, et al., p. 370; Weinstock & Neides, p. 153).

2. **(d)** The fatigue and neurological symptoms reported, and the laboratory results given, suggest that Margaret Green has a vitamin B_{12} deficiency anemia; the serum iron and folic acid levels are within normal limits, but the B_{12} level is low. To determine whether her vitamin B_{12} deficiency is due to dietary deficiencies or GI absorption problems (pernicious anemia), a Schilling test would be drawn. The Schilling test is recommended when a serum vitamin B_{12} level is less than 200 pg/mL. Serum ferritin is useful in differentiating between iron deficiency anemia and anemia of chronic disease; it is one of the earliest changes associated with iron deficiency anemia. The red blood cell folate level is considered more reliable and has replaced serum folate as the appropriate test to document folic acid deficiency anemia and the direct Coombs test is used to diagnose autoimmune hemolytic anemia (Tierney, et al., pp. 371, 487, 495; Wells, et al., 370-371; Weinstock & Neides, pp. 151-152).

3. **(b)** Vitamin B_{12} anemia would be treated with IM injection replacement therapy. The replacement is done by injection since the B_{12} may not be well absorbed in the GI tract. A number of varying vitamin B_{12} replacement protocols are used (Tierney, et al., p. 487; Wells, et al., pp. 372-373; Weinstock & Neides, p. 155).

4. **(c)** Anemia from acute blood loss would be normocytic. The MCV would be in the range of 80 to 100 μ^3 (Little, p. 180; Wells, et al., p. 368).

5. **(b)** The most common cause of iron deficiency anemia in a young middle aged male is gastrointestinal blood loss (Goroll, p. 448; Little, p. 177; Tierney, et al., p. 480; Weinstock & Neides, p. 153).

6. **(a)** Iron deficiency anemia is a microcytic anemia. The only microcytic anemia on this list is thalassemia (Goroll, p. 449; Weinstock & Neides, p. 151; Wells, et al., p. 368).

7. **(d)** The most definitive tests for hemoglobin abnormalities are hemoglobin electrophoresis and peripheral blood smear for morphology. The RDW can be used to distinguish between thalassemia trait and iron deficiency anemia (the RDW is normal in thalassemia trait and increased in iron deficiency), but the erythropoietin level is not considered a useful diagnostic test in mild degrees of anemia, as in this case (Stobo, et al., pp. 703-705; Little, p. 178).

8. **(d)** Folate or folic acid supplementation in women of child bearing age, and during pregnancy, is a preventive measure to reduce the risk of abnormal neural tube development in the fetus (Little, p. 183; USPS Task Force, pp. 1, 874).

9. **(c)** Chemotherapeutic agents, ethanol/alcohol, and a number of drugs (including methotrexate, phenytoin, and phenobarbital which have a frequent incidence of reported megaloblastosis) can cause megaloblastic, or macrocytic, anemias—particularly folate deficiency. Lead toxicity and sickle cell anemia are potential causes of microcytic anemia, while renal failure more typically causes a normocytic anemia of chronic illness (Goroll, p. 431; Little, pp. 180, 182; Wells, et al., pp. 368-369; Weinstock & Neides, p. 153).

10. **(c)** A "shift to the left" commonly occurs in the WBC count in response to bacterial infections. The "left shift" involves: (a) leukocytosis (elevated white blood cell counts) occurring because of the mobilization of granulocytes and/or lymphocytes to ingest and destroy invading organisms, (b) granulocytosis/neutrophilia (elevated neutrophils and basophil counts) occurring as neutrophil production is increased in response to the loss of granulocytes in the mobilization/phagocytic process, and (c) immature forms of neutrophils (bands and segs) are seen on peripheral blood smear as a result of the increased rate of neutrophil production. In a "left shift" WBC counts are usually above 11,000 as in options "c" and "d," neutrophil counts are 60% higher, as in option "c," and seg and band forms of neutrophils are > 10% to 12% (Stobo, et al., p. 734; Wells, et al., p. 398).

11. **(b)** Pregnancy causes increased requirements for iron, and the symptoms of fatigue, shortness of breath on exertion, and pica (the desire to eat substances such as ice or clay) are characteristic symptoms of iron deficiency anemia (as well as pregnancy) (Goroll, p. 448; Tierney, et al., p. 480; Weinstock & Neides, p. 151).

12. **(a)** In the treatment of iron deficiency anemia, therapeutic doses of iron should elevate the reticulocyte count (reticulocytosis) within 7 to 10 days of beginning treatment, indicating that the replacement iron is available and being used to increase red blood cell production (Wells, et al., p. 374).

13. **(c)** Severe dysplasia or carcinoma in situ is CIN III (Weinstock & Neides, p. 53).

14. **(d)** Late age of first live birth, not early age, is a risk factor for breast cancer (USPS Task Force, p. 74; Wells, et al., p. 731).

15. **(b)** Men between the ages of 20 and 40 are at highest risk for testicular cancer; testicular cancer is the most common solid neoplasm in young men between ages 20 and 34 (Stobo, et al., p. 794; USPS Task Force, p. 153).

16. **(a)** In the U.S., African-American women and women of low socioeconomic status have a higher risk of cervical cancer, as do women who smoke, have a history of multiple sexual partners or sexually transmitted diseases, began having sex at an early age, or have had many pregnancies (Stobo, et al., p. 787; USPS Task Force, p. 105).

17. **(a)** Hypercalcemia of malignancy most commonly occurs due to humoral abnormalities triggered by malignancy, or skeletal invasion by tumor. Squamous cell carcinomas of lung, head, and neck, hematologic malignancies such as multiple myeloma or T-cell lymphomas, and carcinomas of breast, ovary, kidney, and bladder are most frequently involved (Stobo, et al., p. 314; Wells, et al., p. 960).

18. **(a)** Uremia causes a platelet disorder that can lead to prolonged bleeding times and anemia secondary to decreased erythropoietin production, while all the rest of the body states or diseases listed can cause hypercoagulatory abnormalities (Stobo, et al., pp. 757-758; Wells, et al., p. 991).

19. **(c)** Trimethoprim/sulfamethoxazole, along with other antimicrobials (including the quinolones, macrolides, tetracyclines, and metronidazole), cimetidine, and gemfibrozil can increase the PT/INR when used with warfarin (Craig & Stitzel, p. 274; Weinstock & Neides p. 183).

20. **(a)** Meperidine is not recommended for the long term management of cancer pain, because its short duration of action (2.5 to 3.5 hours), and its toxic metabolite (normeperidine) which can accumulate and cause CNS stimulation that may lead to seizures. Morphine is actually the standard, most commonly used opioid analgesic for long term cancer pain treatment. All of the other statements are correct, according to the AHCPR guidelines for management of cancer pain in adults (USDHHS & AHCPR, pp. 662-665; Wells, et al., pp. 662-665).

References

Craig, C. R., & Stitzel, R. E. (1997). *Modern pharmacology with clinical applications* (5th ed.). Boston: Little, Brown & Co.

Goroll, A. H., May, L. A., & Mulley, A. G. (1995). *Primary care medicine* (3rd ed.). Philadelphia: J. B. Lippincott.

Little, D. R. (1997). Diagnosis and management of anemia. *Primary care reports, 3*(20), 175-184.

Stobo, J. D., Hellmann, D. B., Ladenson, P. W., Petty, B. G., & Traill, T. A. (Eds.). (1996). *The principles and practice of medicine.* Stamford, CT: Appleton & Lange.

Tierney, Jr., L. M., McPhee, S. J., & Papadakis, M. A. (1998). *Current medical diagnosis and treatment* (37th ed.). Stamford, CT: Appleton & Lange.

U.S. Department of Health and Human Services, (USDHHS) Agency for Health Care Policy and Research (AHCPR). (1994). *Quick reference guide for clinicians Number 9: Management of cancer pain: Adults.* Washington, DC: Government Printing Office.

U.S. Preventive Services (USPS) Task Force. (1996). *Guide to clinical preventive services* (2nd ed.). Baltimore: Williams & Wilkins.

Wells, B. G., DiPiro, J. T., Schwinghammer, T. L., & Hamilton, C.W. (1998). *Pharmacotherapy handbook.* Stamford, CT: Appleton & Lange.

Weinstock, M. B., & Neides, D. M. (1996). *The resident's guide to ambulatory care* (2nd ed.). Columbus, OH: Anadem Publishing.

Gastrointestinal Disorders

Sharon Fruh

Select one best answer to the following questions.

Questions 1, 2, and 3 refer to the following scenario.

Mrs. Smith, a new patient, states that she has been bothered more than usual for the past three months with esophageal burning after meals, a bitter taste in her mouth, and occasional regurgitation of her food.

1. Based on the history described, what is the most likely diagnosis?

    a. Gastroesophageal reflux disease
    b. Esophageal stricture
    c. Achalasia disease
    d. Cancer of the esophagus

2. Which one of the following medications may aggravate Mrs. Smith's condition?

    a. Antacid tablets
    b. Theophylline
    c. Cimetidine
    d. Ampicillin

3. Which of the following is not considered a risk factor for Mrs. Smith's condition?

    a. Cigarette smoking
    b. Excessive alcohol
    c. High coffee intake
    d. Female gender

4. A 52-year-old male executive presents for a routine physical examination. You plan to do a rectal examination as part of the physical examination. You also plan to test for fecal occult blood. Fecal occult blood screening is recommended every:

    a. Year
    b. Five years
    c. Six years
    d. Ten years

Questions 5 and 6 refer to the following scenario.

John Reed, a 56-year-old construction worker who has smoked two packs of cigarettes per day for the past 30 years, is complaining of gnawing and burning epigastric pain occurring 1 to 3 hours after meals. This condition is somewhat relieved by antacids. He awakens in the early morning hours with epigastric pain. He describes dyspepsia. On physical examination, the only significant finding is epigastric tenderness. Laboratory/procedure results indicate a *Helicobacter pylori* infection.

5. The most likely diagnosis based on the above information is:

    a. Cholecystitis
    b. Zollinger-Ellison syndrome
    c. Crohn's disease
    d. Duodenal ulcer

6. What is the treatment of choice for this patient?

    a. Prostaglandins
    b. Antimuscarinic agents
    c. Nonsteroidal anti-iflammatory agents
    d. Triple therapy

Questions 7 and 8 refer to the following scenario.

Mrs. Eagle, a 32-year-old obese Native-American with type 2 diabetes, presents with right upper quadrant discomfort which radiates to her back. She has experienced increasing nausea with vomiting on and off over the last few months. Physical examination reveals localized right upper quadrant tenderness.

7. Based on the above information, what is the tentative diagnosis?

    a. Cirrhosis

b. Viral hepatitis
c. Cholelithiasis
d. Adenomyomatosis

8. Based on your tentative diagnosis, what disease is Mrs. Eagle at risk for developing?

   a. Acute pancreatitis
   b. Chronic pancreatitis
   c. Polyposis syndrome
   d. Gardner's syndrome

Questions 9 and 10 refer to the following scenario.

Sue Anderson, an 18-year-old college student, presents with sharp, right lower quadrant abdominal tenderness. The pain is like a steady ache and increases when she walks or coughs. She has a low grade temperature and is experiencing intermittent vomiting. Physical examination reveals positive psoas and obturator signs. The laboratory reports a WBC of 15,000 mm^3 with neutrophilia.

9. Based on the above information, the most probable diagnosis is:

   a. Irritable bowel syndrome
   b. Ulcerative colitis
   c. Appendicitis
   d. Intestinal tuberculosis

10. Based on the tentative diagnosis for Sue Anderson, the next step would be to:

    a. Suggest a clear liquid diet for 1 to 2 days progressing to bland
    b. Order ampicillin 500 mg orally every six hours
    c. Prescribe bedrest to promote colon rest until symptoms reside
    d. Refer her to a physician for an evaluation

11. Mr. Ashton recently moved to the area. He states that he is here today for a follow-up stool culture. He does not remember what condition he had but, six months ago he had repeated bouts of diarrhea, abdominal cramps, headache, and fever. He states that they found something on his stool culture and told him to return at five months and at one year for repeat cultures. He does not have medical records, but says he was not given antibiotics during his illness. Based on the above history, what was the most probable diagnosis six months ago?

    a. Salmonella
    b. Campylobacter
    c. Shigella
    d. Giardia

12. Before Mrs. Shaw travels to East Africa (high risk destination), what two vaccinations should she receive as her hepatitis prophylaxis treatment?

    a. Hepatitis A and B
    b. Hepatitis B and C
    c. Hepatitis C and D
    d. Hepatitis E and G

13. Which of the following is not a mode of transmission of hepatitis B?

    a. Parenteral
    b. Sexual transmission
    c. Vertical transmission
    d. Oral ingestion

14. When treating an individual with acute hepatitis who cannot keep liquids down, what is an absolute indication for hospital admission?

    a. Prothrombin time > 16 seconds
    b. Elevated liver enzymes
    c. Elevated ferritin level
    d. Elevated BUN

15. Which of the following statements is not true with regard to hepatitis A?

    a. It does not progress to chronic liver disease
    b. Most individuals recover completely
    c. Clinical and biochemical relapses may occur before full recovery
    d. Symptoms occur six weeks to six months following infection

16. Mrs. Nelson, who works at a day care center, was recently diagnosed with hepatitis A. Which of the following statements is true regarding hepatitis A?

    a. Hepatitis A tends to last longer and be more severe than hepatitis B
    b. Chronic hepatitis and carrier states are associated with hepatitis A
    c. Of those patients with hepatitis A, 50% will develop chronic hepatitis
    d. Hepatitis A often presents with nonspecific "flu" like symptoms

Questions 17 and 18 refer to the following scenario.

Mr. James, a 38-year-old client, states that both of his parents had severe diverticulitis. He is worried that he will develop diverticulitis. Mr. James asks what the risk factors for colonic diverticulitis are.

17. Which of the following types of diets place him at high risk of developing this disease?

    a. Low fiber, high fat
    b. High fiber, high fat
    c. Vegetarian
    d. Lactose free

18. Which of the following clinical findings is not typically associated with acute diverticulitis?

    a. Tender abdomen
    b. Low grade temperature
    c. Tender discrete mass
    d. Positive Bernstein test

Questions 19, 20, and 21 refer to the following scenario.

Penny, a 23-year-old graduate student, presents with abdominal pain. She has had this pain for four weeks. She has had episodes of diarrhea alternating with constipation. This started around the time she had midterm examinations. Her physical examination reveals no abnormal findings.

19. Which one of the following treatments would not be recommended for her condition?

    a. Amoxicillin
    b. Psyllium
    c. Dicyclomine
    d. Propantheline

20. Which of the following dietary recommendations would not be appropriate for Penny?

    a. Increase fiber in her diet
    b. Avoid spicy meals
    c. Begin a low calorie diet
    d. Schedule regular meals

21. With regard to Penny's condition, which of the following is not an expected course of this condition?

    a. Recurrences are common
    b. Frequency lessens with increasing age
    c. Stress precipitates episodes
    d. Progression to cancer is a risk

Questions 22 and 23 refer to the following scenario.

A 19-year-old black male complains of abdominal distention and explosive, watery diarrhea after he eats ice cream. His physical examination is unremarkable.

22. What is the appropriate treatment plan for this patient?

    a. Antimotility agents
    b. Antibiotic therapy
    c. Lactose free diet
    d. Barley free diet

23. What is a possible complication of this condition?

    a. Calcium deficiency
    b. Mineral deficiency
    c. Sodium deficiency
    d. Potassium deficiency

Answers and Rationale

1. **(a)** In gastroesophageal reflux disease (GERD), heartburn is present in 70% to 85% of patients, regurgitation 60%, and bitter taste in mouth 50%. With esophageal stricture, the presenting symptom is dysphagia, more often with solids than liquids. Achalasia is a relatively rare disease (this patient has dysphagia with solids and liquids, and heartburn is a rare complaint). Cancer of the esophagus is rare (Nobel, pp. 587-595).

2. **(b)** The following medications lower esophageal pressure: Theophylline, anticholinergics, progesterone, calcium channel blockers, alpha adrenergic agents, diazepam, and meperidine. Gastroesophageal reflux should be considered in the differential diagnosis of adult onset asthma (Nobel, pp. 587-595).

3. **(d)** Males and females are equally affected (Nobel, pp. 587-595).

4. **(a)** The U.S. Preventive Services Task Force currently recommends annual screening for fecal occult blood in asymptomatic patients over age 50 (USPS Task Force, p. 46-53).

5. **(d)** 90% to 95% of duodenal ulcers are caused by *H. pylori* (Tierney, et al., p. 577).

6. **(d)** Triple antibiotic therapy is currently recommended to eradicate the *Helicobacter pylori* (Rakel, 1998, p. 528).

7. **(c)** The clinical finding of gallstones is present only during an acute gallbladder attack. Examination reveals epigastric and right upper quadrant tenderness. Gallstones are more common in women than in men. Native-Americans have a high rate of cholesterol cholelithiasis, perhaps due to a genetic predisposition. Obesity is a risk factor for gallstones. The incidence is increased in individuals with diabetes mellitus (Tierney, et al., pp. 652-657).

8. **(a)** The two most common causes of acute pancreatitis are alcohol use and gallstones (Bergin, pp. 280, 285).

9. **(c)** The symptoms described are classic. Appendicitis is the most common abdominal surgical emergency, affecting approximately 10% of the population (Tierney, et al., p. 600).

10. **(d)** Refer all individuals with suspected or diagnosed appendicitis to a physician and/or a surgeon (Rakel, 1996, p. 369).

11. **(a)** The above symptoms are classic for salmonella. The repeated stools are to diagnose chronic carriers. All of the other conditions listed require antibiotics; however, with salmonella, antibiotics have no benefits and prolong the carrier state (Rakel, 1996, pp. 858-861).

12. **(a)** Hepatitis A and B vaccines are currently used to protect high risk individuals, including travelers, from these diseases. There are no vaccinations available for the hepatitis C, D, E, and G viruses (Rakel, 1996, p. 369).

13. **(d)** Hepatitis B is not transmitted via oral ingestion (Rakel, 1998, p. 491).

14. **(a)** The best immediate measure of the liver's ability to function is the prothrombin time. The severity of liver injury can only be assessed by evaluating the prothrombin time. Liver enzymes can remain elevated for a period of time and do not give an indication of the immediate function of the liver (Dambro, p. 462).

15. **(d)** Options "a," "b," and "c" are true with regard to hepatitis A, however, the onset of symptoms is two to six weeks following infection (Tierney, et al., p. 635).

16. **(d)** Hepatitis A most commonly presents with "flu" like symptoms. It is generally a mild hepatitis and does not lead to a carrier or chronic state (Nobel, pp. 614-619).

17. **(a)** A low fiber and high fat diet slows the rate at which food passes through the intestine (Rakel, 1996, p. 352).

18. **(d)** A tender abdomen, discrete mass, and low grade temperature are common

findings in diverticulitis. A positive Bernstein test is commonly found in gastroesophageal reflux disease (Rakel, 1996, p. 299, 351).

19. **(a)** Antibiotics are not indicated for irritable bowel syndrome. Increase in fiber and anticholinergic and antispasmodic agents are helpful (Rudy & Kurowski, p. 233).

20. **(c)** A low calorie diet is not included in the routine treatment for irritable bowel syndrome (Rudy & Kurowski, p. 233).

21. **(d)** Irritable bowel syndrome does not place individuals at risk for cancer (Rudy & Kurowski, p. 233).

22. **(c)** This individual has lactose intolerance. Reducing or restricting dietary lactose can control symptoms. Commercially available "lactase" preparations are often effective in reducing symptoms in individuals (Bergin, p. 253).

23. **(a)** When individuals totally avoid all dairy products they are at risk for a possible calcium deficiency. Taking lactase prior to ingesting milk products can be helpful in assuring they receive an adequate amount of calcium. Sometimes yogurt and fermented products such as hard cheeses are tolerated. Supplemental calcium is also recommended (Bergin, p. 253).

References

Bergin, J. D. (1997). *Medicine recall.* Baltimore: Williams & Wilkins.

Dambro, M. R. (1997). *Griffith's 5 minute clinical consult.* Baltimore: Williams & Wilkins.

Noble, J. (Ed.). (1996). *Textbook of primary care medicine.* (2nd ed.). St. Louis: Mosby.

Rakel, R. E. (1998). *Conn's current therapy.* Philadelphia: W. B. Saunders.

Rakel, R. E. (1996). *Saunders manual of medical practice.* Philadelphia: W. B. Saunders.

Rudy, D. R., & Kurowski, K. (1997). *Family medicine.* Baltimore: Williams & Wilkins.

Tierney, L. M., Jr., McPhee, S. J., & Papadakis, M. A. (1998). *Current medical diagnosis and treatment* (37th ed.). Stamford, CT: Appleton & Lange.

U.S. Preventive Services (USPS) Task Force. (1996). *Guide to clinical preventive services* (2nd ed.). Baltimore: Williams & Wilkins.

Endocrine Disorders

Sharon Fruh

Select one best answer to the following questions.

1. A new patient, Mrs. Lizaragra, age 44, has recently had a physical examination for a new employment opportunity. Her history was unremarkable. Physical examination revealed that she was approximately 20% over her ideal body weight. Her laboratory results were within normal limits except for her fasting blood sugar which was 138 mg/dL. Based on the above information, recommendation for return follow-up would be:

    a. As needed since she is essentially healthy
    b. One year for a repeat of her fasting blood sugar
    c. Six months for a repeat of her fasting blood sugar
    d. Within one week to repeat her fasting blood sugar

Questions 2 and 3 refer to the following scenario.

2. Mr. Creekwood, a 42-year-old Native American, has been recently diagnosed with hypertension. Both of his parents have type 2 diabetes. Physical examination revealed that he is 30% above his ideal body weight and has a large waist-hip ratio. These findings are suggestive of:

    a. Diabetes insipidus
    b. Syndrome X
    c. Sjogren's syndrome
    d. Hashimoto's thyroiditis

3. The best disease prevention measures for Mr. Creekwood include which of the following?

    a. Increase potassium consumption
    b. Fluid replacement
    c. Levothyroxine

d. Weight loss and exercise

Questions 4, 5, and 6 refer to the following scenario.

Mrs. Jones presents with a variety of symptoms including weakness, weight loss, and palpitations. Physical examination reveals that she has eyelid retraction and an enlarged thyroid gland. Auscultation of the thyroid gland reveals a systolic bruit, and a thrill is palpable.

4. Based on the above information, the nurse practitioner should suspect:

   a. Primary hypothyroidism
   b. Graves' disease
   c. Myxedema
   d. Thyroid nodule

5. Which of the following laboratory results would be unexpected in Mrs. Jones' evaluation?

   a. Suppressed TSH
   b. Elevated total T_4, T_3 resin uptake
   c. Elevated free T_4 and/or T_3
   d. Normal free T_4 and elevated TSH

6. Which of the following treatments would be appropriate for Mrs. Jones?

   a. Levothyroxine
   b. Prednisone
   c. Insulin
   d. Propylthiouracil

7. Mrs. Miller has an enlarged thyroid gland. Her TSH levels are elevated. This information makes you suspect that Mrs. Miller has which one of the following conditions?

   a. Subacute thyroiditis
   b. Graves' disease
   c. Hypothyroidism
   d. Thyrotoxicosis

8. A common cause of hyperthyroidism that should always be identified during a thorough history is:

   a. Radiation of the thyroid gland

   b. Ingestion of too much thyroid hormone

   c. A history of type 2 diabetes mellitus

   d. A history of thyroid cysts

9. When assessing an individual from a developing country who has a goiter, it is important to identify if they have a dietary deficiency of:

   a. Mineral

   b. Sodium

   c. Zinc

   d. Iodine

10. A healthy, 32-year-old female presents with atrial fibrillation. Which endocrine disorder should be included in your differential diagnosis?

   a. Hypothyroidism

   b. Thyroid nodules

   c. Hyperthyroidism

   d. Thyroid cancer

11. Hypothyroidism is most difficult to identify in persons aged:

   a. 21 to 30 years

   b. 31 to 50 years

   c. 51 to 60 years

   d. Over 70 years

12. A 52-year-old male with a goiter is concerned that it may be malignant. What age group is at greatest risk for malignancy when a goiter is found?

   a. < 15 and > 70

   b. 20 to 40

   c. 45 to 65

   d. 65 to 70

Questions 13, 14, and 15 refer to the following scenario.

13. Mrs. Ortego, an obese 62-year-old female, has three fasting blood sugars > than 142 mg/dL. Which of the following treatments would place her at risk for lactic acidosis?

   a. Acarbose

   b. Metformin

    c. Sulfonylureas

    d. Troglitazone

14. The decision is made to begin oral antidiabetic treatment. Which of the following oral medications has the greatest potential to precipitate a hypoglycemic episode?

    a. Acarbose

    b. Metformin

    c. Tolbutamide

    d. Troglitazone

15. Mrs. Ortego is at risk for which one of the following conditions?

    a. Cardiovascular disease

    b. Ketoacidosis

    c. Ulcerative colitis

    d. Hypothyroidism

16. Ms. Leo was seen yesterday for a vaginal yeast infection, and during routine screening was found to have a fasting blood sugar of 300 mg/dL. She presents today for full evaluation and treatment plan. Which of the following is least likely to be assessed at this visit?

    a. Glycosylated hemoglobin A_{1c}

    b. Blood glucose

    c. Ocular fundus

    d. Feet

Questions 17, 18, and 19 refer to the following scenario.

Mr. Charles, is an obese, 68-year-old patient with type 2 diabetes controlled on insulin. During his routine diabetes check-up he reported a high fasting glucose in the morning. He does not have nocturnal hypoglycemia. His blood sugars are within normal limits the rest of the day.

17. This would suggest which of the following problems?

    a. NPH insulin allergy

    b. Somogyi effect

    c. Dawn phenomenon

    d. Diabetes honeymoon period

18. Mr. Charles returned a few weeks later stating that he got all mixed up with his medications. He presents with pallor, sweating, and anxiety. Physical examination reveals tachycardia. The ANP would expect Mr. Charles' serum glucose to be:

    a. 20-35 mg/dL
    b. 45-60 mg/dL
    c. 220-260 mg/dL
    d. 400-460 mg/dL

19. What would be the appropriate treatment for Mr. Charles?

    a. Insulin
    b. Oral glucose
    c. Oral hypoglycemic agents
    d. Bicarbonate

20. A 20-year-old female presents for family planning. During the health history she reveals that her mother and maternal grandmother have type 2 diabetes mellitus, and she asks if she should be tested. The ANP replies that:

    a. Screening is recommended only if obese
    b. Screening is recommended for first degree relatives
    c. Type 2 diabetes is more common in females than males
    d. Screening is not recommended under 40 years of age

Questions 21 and 22 refer to the following scenario.

Mrs. Kovik, a 68-year-old accountant, presents with many unusual complaints. She states that over the past six months she has had weight loss, weakness, nausea, vomiting, abdominal pain, salt cravings, and loss of body hair. Physical examination identifies hypotension and hyperpigmentation over her elbows, gingival margins, and under her brassiere straps. Her laboratory results indicate a decreased serum sodium level and an elevated serum potassium level.

21. Based upon the above assessment findings, what diagnosis is most probable for Mrs. Kovik?

    a. Hyperparathyroidism
    b. Cushing's syndrome
    c. Pheochromocytoma
    d. Addison's disease

22. Mrs. Kovik will be referred to a physician. You expect that the cornerstone of her treatment will be:

    a. Calcium
    b. Surgery
    c. Hydrocortisone
    d. Beta blockers

23. June, a 42-year-old patient with type 1 diabetes, has fasting blood sugars which are above 200 mg/dL. The only medication that she is presently taking is insulin. Your next course of action is to:

    a. Add acarbose
    b. Add metformin
    c. Increase her insulin
    d. Add troglitazone

Answers and Rationale

1. **(d)** According to the new (1997) American Diabetes Association Consensus Statement, diagnostic criteria for diagnosing type 2 diabetes mellitus consists of two or more fasting blood sugars above 126 mg/dL. It is important that the individual return within one week to repeat the fasting blood sugar (ADA Clinical Practice Recommendations, pp. 6-10).

2. **(b)** Syndrome X is a constellation of clinical problems including glucose intolerance, hyperinsulinemia (insulin resistance), hyperlipidemia, and hypertension (Bergin, p. 562; Tierney, et al., p. 1072; Nobel, p. 476).

3. **(d)** Weight loss and exercise is the best disease prevention measure (Bergin, p. 562; Nobel, p. 476).

4. **(b)** These are some of the classic symptoms of Graves' disease (Nobel, pp. 498-509).

5. **(d)** A normal free T_4 and mildly increased TSH is found in subclinical hypothyroidism (Rakel, 1998, pp. 636-641).

6. **(d)** Propylthiouracil (PTU) inhibits the conversion of T_4 to T_3 in the periphery (Rakel, 1998, p. 651).

7. **(c)** TSH is elevated in hypothyroidism (Dambro, p. 546).

8. **(b)** Surreptitious prescription or over medication of exogenous thyroid is often seen by the health care professional as a frequent cause of hyperthyroidism (Rakel, 1996, p. 638).

9. **(d)** About 5% of the world's population have goiters. Approximately 75% of these people live in geographic areas that have an iodine deficiency (Tierney, et al., p. 1055).

10. **(c)** Hyperthyroidism can bring about several abnormal cardiac findings including atrial fibrillation, sinus tachycardia, and paroxysmal supraventricular tachycardia (Rakel, 1996, p. 638).

11. **(d)** Symptoms of hypothyroidism in the elderly can often be mistakenly attributed to the aging process (Rudy & Kurowsky, p. 553).

12. **(a)** Less than 15 and greater than 70 years of age are significant in relation to elevated risk for malignancy when a goiter is present (Rakel, 1996, pp. 498-515).

13. **(b)** Metformin has an adverse affect of lactic acidosis (Tierney, et al., p. 1107).

14. **(c)** The sulfonylureas are the only antidiabetic medications that promote insulin release from the pancreas, and as a result may cause hypoglycemia. Acarbose inhibits sucrose cleavage in the gut, metformin inhibits gluconeogenesis, and troglitazone potentiates the action of circulating insulin and decreases hepatic glucose output. Because the medications listec in choices ''a,'' ''b,'' and ''d'' do not increase the amount of circulating insulin, hypoglycemia is not typically a concern (Tierney, et al., pp. 1104-1108).

15. **(a)** Cardiovascular disease is the leading cause of death in patients with diabetes (Rakel, 1998, p. 551).

16. **(a)** Glycosylated hemoglobin A_{1c} documents the level of glycemic control in the previous 120 days. Because this patient is newly diagnosed, her previous control would be poor. The other choices are all baseline assessments that are appropriate for a first visit (Tierney, et al., p. 1119).

17. **(c)** The dawn phenomenon is a state of relative insulin resistance in the early morning hours caused by a variation in the counter-regulatory hormones. This can result in elevated blood glucose levels in the morning with an increased insulin requirement (Tierney, et al., p. 1118).

18. **(b)** This patient is experiencing classic symptoms of hypoglycemia. The most common range of hypoglycemia is 45 to 60 mg/dL. Additionally, if this patient's glucose were in the 20 to 35 g/dL range he would likely be experiencing an altered level of consciousness (Dambro, pp. 530-531).

19. **(b)** When the patient is awake and alert oral glucose is the treatment of choice.

If the patient becomes unresponsive, then should be given 50 cc of 50% glucose IV (Rakel, 1996, p. 638).

20. **(b)** Heredity plays a large role in the pathogenesis of type 2 diabetes mellitus (greater than a 90% concordance between monozygotic twins). Due to her strong family history it is necessary to screen at a younger age and more frequently than in the general population. Options "a," "c," and "d" are not true (Rakel, 1996, pp. 655).

21. **(d)** The symptoms described are classic for Addison's disease (Tierney, et al., pp. 1073-1075).

22. **(c)** Hydrocortisone in the lowest effective dose is the preferred treatment for Addison's disease (Rakel, 1996, p. 655).

23. **(c)** Increasing her insulin is the only option. The other medications are indicated for type 2 diabetes (Tierney, et al., p. 1108-1112).

References

American Diabetes Association Clinical Practice Recommendations. (1997). *Diabetes Care*, 20 (suppl 1).

Bergin, J. D. (1997). *Medicine recall*. Baltimore: Williams & Wilkins.

Dambro, M. R. (1997). *Griffith's 5 minute clinical consult*. Baltimore: Williams & Wilkins.

Nobel, J. (Ed.). (1996). *Textbook of primary care medicine*. (2nd ed.). Philadelphia: W. B. Saunders.

Rakel, R. E. (1998). *Conn's current therapy*. Philadelphia: W. B. Saunders.

Rakel, R. E. (1996). *Saunders manual of medical practice*. Philadelphia: W. B. Saunders.

Rudy, D. R., & Kurowki, K. (1997). *Family medicine*. Baltimore: Williams & Wilkins.

Tierney, Jr., L. M., McPhee, S. J., & Papadakis, M. A. (1998). *Current medical diagnosis and treatment* (37th ed.). Stamford, CT: Appleton & Lange.

Genitourinary and Gynecologic Disorders

Carol Gemberling

Select one best answer to the following questions.

1. A 22-year-old patient tells you that she has had an unusual vaginal discharge for the last week and now she is experiencing vague lower abdominal discomfort. Her new partner of one month has been unfaithful and she has decided to discontinue seeing him because he refuses to use a condom. Her pelvic examination reveals a scant mucopurulent cervical discharge and mild vaginal erythema. There is no cervical motion tenderness or pelvic mass appreciated. Which of the following are the appropriate tests to perform today on this afebrile patient?

    a. Wet prep, herpes titer, and RPR
    b. Gonorrhea and chlamydia cultures, and wet prep
    c. VDRL, KOH evaluation, and hepatitis B titer
    d. General bacterial culture, cervical biopsy, and Pap smear

2. The vaginal culture of a young woman is positive for chlamydia. Which of the following is the current drug of choice for this condition?

    a. Ampicillin
    b. Doxycycline
    c. Erythromycin
    d. Sulfisoxazole

3. Sexually active women need specific counseling regarding their risk of contracting sexually transmitted infections. Which of the following statements best reflects current information regarding chlamydia infections?

    a. Women in the 20 to 40 year age group are most commonly diagnosed with chlamydia

b. Untreated patients can later present with single, large joint septic arthritis, fever, and elevated WBC count

c. Warty growths can appear on the cervix in women who are untreated

d. Sequelae include infertility, ectopic pregnancies, and urethral syndromes

Questions 4 and 5 refer to the following scenario.

You are the ANP working in a college student health service and your 20-year-old patient tells you that she has noticed some painless "bumps down there." Upon further exploration, she tells you that recently her boyfriend was seen in the student health care center and was told that he had a virus infection that was transmitted sexually. The remainder of the history and physical are negative for previous sexually transmitted infection or abnormal pelvic finding except for the multiple 2 to 4 mm raised, warty growths.

4. Which diagnosis is most likely?

a. Herpes simplex
b. Syphilis
c. Human papillomavirus
d. Lymphogranuloma venereum *vesicular or ulcerative lesion on external genitalia c̄ inguinal lymphadenitis or BUBOES.*

5. Current therapeutic recommendations for the above infection would include which of the following?

a. Application of trichloroacetic acid or podofilox directly on the lesion
b. Biopsy for typing of the lesion before initiating treatment
c. Betadine douches every other day for one to two weeks
d. Sulfa vaginal cream twice a day for seven days

6. While performing a gynecologic examination you are careful to obtain an adequate sampling for the Pap smear. Which of the following areas is the most likely site for cervical cancer to originate?

a. Internal cervical os
b. External cervical os
c. Mucoepithelial junction
d. Transformation zone

7. Ms. Highland is a 25-year-old teacher being seen for increasing vaginal odor and mild vulvovaginal inflammation, especially after intercourse. She is using

oral contraceptives and occasionally uses condoms with her fiance. While performing your pelvic examination you identify a fishy odor that becomes more apparent when you are performing your wet prep for microscopic evaluation. Which best reflects your diagnostic suspicion?

- a. Candida vaginitis
- b. Atrophic vaginitis
- c. Bacterial vaginosis
- d. Retained tampon

8. While working in student health at a local community college, a female patient complains of vaginal discharge, itching, vulvovaginal irritation and dysuria. She has recently completed a seven day course of over-the-counter antifungal vaginal cream, but reports that this has not improved her symptoms. Her partner was recently treated for an infection with a medication that was to be taken while abstaining from alcohol ingestion. She and her partner use condoms sporadically. On pelvic examination you find a malodorous frothy green discharge with strawberry spots on the vagina and cervix. Which of the following conditions is the most likely etiology?

- a. Herpes simples virus
- b. Trichomonas vaginitis
- c. Candida vaginitis
- d. Chlamydia vaginitis

9. A 19-year-old female patient has complaints of bilateral lower abdominal and pelvic discomfort that is worse during intercourse. She feels as if she might have a slight fever and began having chills this morning. She denies any increase in vaginal discharge or odor and is unaware of any symptoms in her partner. Upon physical examination she has a temperature of 101° F, abdominal and cervical motion tenderness, and mucopurulent cervical discharge. Which of the following organisms must you cover in your antibiotic therapy?

- a. *Mycoplasma hominis, C. trachomatis,* anaerobes, and *N. gonorrhoeae*
- b. *T. pallidum, Haemophilus ducreyi,* aerobes, and *Mycoplasma hominis*
- c. *C. glabrata, C. tropicalis,* anerobes, and *C. trachomatis*
- d. *Trichomonas vaginalis, N. gonorrhoeae,* aerobes, and *C. glabrata*

10. The diagnosis of pelvic inflammatory disease is generally made by clinical findings. Which three clinical findings should be present in order to accurately diagnose pelvic inflammatory disease?

a. Gram stain of cervical discharge showing gram negative diplococci, fever, and adnexal tenderness

b. Direct abdominal tenderness, cervical or uterine motion tenderness, and adnexal tenderness

c. Serous fluid from the peritoneal cavity on culdocentesis or laparoscopy, and leukocytosis greater than 20,000 mm^3

d. Nausea and vomiting, adnexal tenderness, and a gram stain showing gram positive extracellular diplococci

Questions 11, 12, and 13 refer to the following scenario.

Ms. Windstone is a 23-year-old with a one day history of frequency, urgency, and dysuria. Other relevant history includes two previous urinary tract infections (UTI) at age 19 after she first became sexually active. She has recently started a new sexual relationship and has had an increased frequency of coitus for the past week. She denies fever, chills, flank or abdominal pain, vaginal discharge or lesions. Physical examination findings include a temperature of 98.4° F, BP of 110/60 mm Hg, no costovertebral angle (CVA) tenderness, and mild suprapubic tenderness. She has no known allergies and takes no medications except oral contraceptives. Vulva is without lesions, and examination of Bartholin's glands, urethra, and Skene's glands reveal no discharge or apparent urethral-hymenal fusion. Urinalysis on an unspun midstream specimen is positive for WBCs, RBCs, and nitrites, but negative for glucose and protein. The pH is 6. Microscopic evaluation yields 10 WBC/HPF, 2 to 3 RBC/HPF, 3 to 5 epithelial cells, and moderate motile bacteria.

11. Which of the following is your most likely diagnosis?

    a. Pyelonephritis
    b. Acute urethral syndrome
    c. Acute uncomplicated cystitis
    d. Recurrent UTI

12. Ms. Windstone expresses concern regarding the recurrence of her symptoms after several years of being symptom free. Which of the following most likely caused the recurrence?

    a. Recent increase in sexual frequency
    b. Oral contraceptives
    c. Abnormalities of the urinary tract
    d. Nephrolithiasis

13. The most appropriate medication regimen for Ms. Windstone would be which one of the following?

    a. Norfloxacin
    b. Erythromycin
    c. Metronidazole
    d. Trimethoprim/sulfamethoxazole

14. Which of the following statements best reflects current thinking with regard to the diagnosis and management of urinary tract infections in an adult male population?

    a. Single dose or short course therapy is generally useful in bacteriuric men
    b. *Escherichia coli* is responsible for approximately 75% of infections in men
    c. A urine culture should be obtained for all men with symptoms suggesting a UTI
    d. Gram positive bacilli cause the majority of UTI in men

15. Which of the following statements is true regarding urinary tract infections in males?

    a. The incidence is highest in infants and elderly hospitalized or institutionalized men
    b. UTI is rarely associated with the onset of sexual activity or the use of condoms
    c. Circumcision is not considered to be a factor in the incidence of UTI
    d. The incidence of asymptomatic bacteriuria is approximately 10% in young men

16. While performing a pelvic examination on your 39-year-old African-American patient, you palpate a painless, asymmetric uterine contour. Your patient is asymptomatic and denies a personal or family history of gynecologic cancers, or abnormal uterine bleeding. Which of the following diagnosis should you suspect?

    a. Endometriosis
    b. Endometrial cancer
    c. Leiomyoma
    d. Adenomyosis

17. Upon examination of your 64-year-old male patient's prostate you feel an abnormality which you suspect is a sign of prostate cancer. Which of the following signs and symptoms is most suggestive of early prostate cancer?

    a. Dysuria, hesitancy, and a boggy prostate
    b. Unilateral, tender testicle with urinary frequency
    c. Hard nodules of the prostate with lumbosacral spine pain
    d. Subtle consistency changes in the prostate without urinary symptoms

18. Which statement best describes factors which put a female patient at the greatest risk for developing breast cancer?

    a. First degree relative with bilateral, premenopausal breast cancer
    b. Personal history of bilateral, fibrocyctic breast changes
    c. Early menarche, late menopause, or late age of first childbirth
    d. Use of oral contraceptives or hormone replacement therapy

Questions 19 and 20 refer to the following scenario.

A 56-year-old patient is being evaluated for a left breast lump which she discovered three months ago while showering. She reports that it seems to be getting smaller but she is not sure and wants you to evaluate it more thoroughly. She last had a mammogram when she turned 50 and has not returned for annual evaluations. Upon careful inspection and palpation of the breast and surrounding lymph nodes, you are able to palpate a 1 cm soft, slightly tender, well circumscribed, round mass in the upper outer quadrant. A similar but smaller mirror image mass is located in the right breast.

19. Which one of the following plans is most appropriate for this patient?

    a. Have her return for evaluation of the masses in one month to assure they are regressing
    b. Schedule her for a mammogram and have her return in one month for a follow-up evaluation
    c. Schedule her for a fine needle aspiration and an ultrasound of the left breast mass
    d. Refer her for an open biopsy with a breast surgeon

20. At your patient's follow-up visit, you note that the bilateral breast masses have disappeared and her most recent mammogram is negative. Based upon these clinical and diagnostic findings, you conclude that your patient probably had

cysts associated with fibrocystic breast changes. Which of the following statements best reflects our current knowledge of this condition?

    a. Fibrocystic changes greatly increase a woman's risk for breast cancer some time in her life

    b. Fibrocystic changes require the same frequency of follow-up as ductal carcinoma in situ

    c. Fibrocystic changes require frequent ultrasound guided biopsies in order to rule out cancer

    d. Nonproliferative fibrocystic changes do not increase a woman's risk of breast cancer

Questions 21 and 22 refer to the following scenario.

Mr. Stowell is a 30-year-old patient who was recently diagnosed with HIV, and is doing very well on antiretroviral therapy. He presents today for his annual examination and update of his immunizations. He had a tetanus booster three years ago when he lacerated his finger, but has not received any other immunizations since childhood. He remembers having measles as a child but does not recall having any other childhood diseases.

21. Which of the following statements best describes the immunizations he needs to receive today or in the near future?

    a. Pneumococcal vaccine, Haemophilus influenza type b vaccine, influenza vaccine, and serology for antibodies to hepatitis B

    b. Influenza vaccine, Bacille Calmette-Guerin (BCG) vaccine, pneumococcal vaccine, and serology for herpes simplex virus titer

    c. Measles, mumps, and rubella (MMR), live oral polio, *Haemophilus influenzae,* and serology for Epstein-Barr virus titer

    d. BCG vaccine, live oral polio vaccine, MMR, and the first in a series of three hepatitis B vaccines

22. During your follow-up visit with Mr. Stowell you review the common sites of opportunistic infections, and the signs and symptoms to which he should be alert. Which of the following statements best reflects the systems or body locations most seriously affected by opportunistic infections in patients with HIV?

    a. Cardiac, musculoskeletal, and auditory

    b. Gastrointestinal, genitourinary, and oral

    c. Neurologic, pulmonary, and gastrointestinal

    d. Dermatologic, reproductive, and endocrine

Answers and Rationale

1. **(b)** The most common causes of vaginitis are infections, including bacterial vaginosis, candidiasis, and trichomoniasis. Exposure to STD is common and women are often asymptomatic. Chlamydia, trichomoniasis, and gonorrhea are the three most prevalent and should be tested for in this client. An HIV test is a good idea as well even though the actual incidence is much lower than the other conditions listed above (Rosenfeld, pp. 383-397, 491-502).

2. **(b)** Several treatment regimes are therapeutic, but this agent is the drug of choice in a nonpregnant and nonallergic individual (Rosenfeld, p. 385).

3. **(d)** Chlamydia has a predilection for the fallopian tubes and 75% of female patients are asymptomatic. PID, infertility, dyspareunia, postcoital bleeding, lower abdominal pain, dysfunctional uterine bleeding, cervicitis, and urethral syndromes are common sequelae of untreated chlamydia (Rosenfeld, pp. 383-392).

4. **(c)** This client demonstrates the typical presentation of the human papillomavirus infection. The fact that her partner has similar growths, was told that he had a virus infection, that the lesions are painless and multiple, and that HPV is the fourth most common STD infection leads us to make this diagnosis. Herpes, syphilis, and lymphogranuloma venereum are the sixth, eighth, and eleventh most common causes of sexually transmitted infection reported in the United States (Rosenfeld, pp. 383-397).

5. **(a)** Despite the fact that there are many good treatment options available to treat HPV, the only appropriate therapeutic choice seen in this question is the application of TCA or podofilox. Some clinicians do not treat small asymptomatic lesions, but many feel that therapy may be initiated primarily for cosmetic reasons as the virus is never completely eradicated (Tierney, et al., p. 695).

6. **(d)** When the transformation zone is not sampled, the sample frequently is returned with the classification of "satisfactory for evaluation but limited by. . . . " The specimen is judged satisfactorily adequate, or not, when it is evaluated. Satisfactory has both endocervical and metaplastic ectocervical

cells easily visible and no more than 50% of the cells obscured by inflammation, blood, or debris (Rosenfeld, p. 457).

7. **(c)** Clinical features of bacterial vaginosis include malodorous, profuse discharge that is thin, homogenous, and gray/white or has a yellow/green tint. Women often complain of increased discharge after intercourse or at the time of menses, and may describe a fishy odor. In order to test for the presence of this odor, the amine test can be performed by adding 10% KOH to a sample of vaginal secretions. A fishy odor predicts vaginosis with 95% reliability (Rosenfeld, pp. 496-497).

8. **(b)** Trichomonas vaginitis exhibits a variety of symptoms compared to other causes of vaginitis. This organism can be asymptomatic in up to 50% of women for long periods of time. The most common symptoms are vaginal discharge, pruritis, vulvovaginal irritation, dyspareunia and dysuria. On assessment, frothy yellow or green discharge may be seen with "strawberry vagina" and significant vaginal erythema (Rosenfeld, pp. 498-499).

9. **(a)** The organisms listed are currently the most prevalent and frequent causes of PID. Other pathogens listed cause syphilis, lymphogranuloma venereum, candida vaginitis, and trichomonas vaginitis (Rosenfeld, pp. 384-395, 492-499).

10. **(b)** The woman must present with three symptoms in order to make the diagnosis of PID. These include direct abdominal tenderness, tenderness with motion of the cervix and uterus, and adnexal tenderness. Besides these three she must have one of the following: Gram-negative intracellular diplococci, temperature greater that 98.4° F, leukocytosis greater than 10,000 mm^3, purulent material from the peritoneal cavity, or pelvic abscess, induration, or mass (Tierney, et al., p. 704).

11. **(c)** Acute uncomplicated UTI, which includes acute dysuria, acute cystitis, and acute urethral syndrome, occurs in otherwise healthy women with structurally and functionally normal urinary tracts. In approximately 70% of women, an acute UTI affects only the bladder and/or urethra. Symptoms include urinary frequency, burning, urgency, and often suprapubic discomfort; flank pain and fever are rare. Recurrent infection implies relapse after treatment of the initial UTI, usually within six weeks, but generally within

1 to 2 weeks following cessation of antibiotic therapy. Uncomplicated py-elonephritis occurs when the soft tissues of the kidney are infected. Uncom-plicated pyelonephritis includes systemic symptoms such as fever, rigors, sweats, headache, nausea and vomiting, malaise, prostration, flank, and low back or abdominal pain, along with lower tract symptoms. Complicated UTI implies the presence of conditions such as sustained repeated infec-tions, inflammatory changes, stones, or obstruction or neurological lesions interfering with the drainage of urine in some part of the urinary tract (Ro-senfeld, pp. 707-718).

12. **(a)** History of recent increase in sexual frequency is one of the most important risk factors for urinary tract infections, presumably from the mechanical ef-fect of introducing pathogens into the bladder (Rosenfeld, pp. 706-709).

13. **(d)** Antibiotics of choice for a nonpregnant woman with an acute uncompli-cated urinary tract infection include amoxicillin, sulfisoxazole, sulfamethox-azole, trimethoprim/sulfamethoxazole, cephalexin, or nitrofuradantoin (Ro-senfeld, pp. 703-713).

14. **(c)** Male UTI is different from those found in women in that *E. coli* is the of-fending organism in only about 25% of the cases, and gram negative bacilli the cause in about 75% of the cases. A urine culture is an important part of diagnosis before any instrumentation. An IVP is indicated as part of the work-up for a male patient with a urinary tract infection. Treatment in men requires longer therapy although the appropriate duration is debatable. Available data suggest that 7 to 10 days of treatment with any one of sev-eral antibiotics is effective for uncomplicated cystitis (Fihn & DeWitt, pp. 596-597).

15. **(a)** In community surveys, the frequency of bacteriuria is age related in men. Prevalence is less than 0.1% in young men and about 15% of those older than age 85. Bacteriuria is found in about 5% of adult male outpatients and in over 25% of elderly hospitalized or institutionalized men. A risk factor in infants and young men is lack of circumcision. Sexual activity appears to predispose to urinary tract infections in men, as does HIV (Fihn & De-Witt, pp. 596-597).

16. **(c)** Leiomyomas are found in 20% of women over age 35, and 30% of these women have abnormal vaginal bleeding. Submucous leiomyomas are most

often associated with abnormal bleeding, given their location just underneath the endometrial layer where they can disrupt the vascular supply to the endometrium. This can result in bleeding secondary to necrosis and ischemia. Tumors in the myometrium (intramural leiomyomas) can distort the uterus and cause pain but are less commonly associated with abnormal bleeding. Endometrial cancer, endometriosis, and adenomyosis are more often associated with abnormal bleeding and/or dysmenorrhea, and pain may be evident with endometriosis depending on the site and severity of involvement (Rosenfeld, pp. 424-429).

17. **(d)** Most early stage malignancies are asymptomatic, and there may be only subtle alterations in the consistency of the prostate. Hard nodules, however, can often be palpated in patients with higher stage disease. Locally advanced prostate cancer can cause irritative and obstructive symptoms, dysuria, and hematuria. Metastatic disease often presents as lumbosacral bone pain, spinal cord compression, unexplained anemia, and weight loss (Fihn & DeWitt, pp. 571-573, 579-580).

18. **(a)** Most of the known risk factors are associated with only mild to moderate increases in risk, but exceptions include a family history of premenopausal carcinoma, or personal history of atypical hyperplasia or carcinoma in situ in breast tissue (Rosenfeld, pp. 684-689).

19. **(b)** This patient is long overdue for a mammogram, and evaluation of masses in postmenopausal women is best done after obtaining a mammogram. Even if the mammogram is negative, further evaluation and follow-up are necessary for a questionable mass (Rosenfeld, pp. 684-692).

20. **(d)** Fibrocystic breast changes comprise a heterogenous group of lesions associated with varying degrees of breast cancer risk. Nonproliferative lesions (cysts, fibrosis, and mild epithelial hyperplasia) are not associated with any increase in breast cancer risk. Proliferative disease without atypia such as papilloma, sclerosing adenosis, and moderate hyperplasia of usual types is associated with a slight increase in breast cancer risk (Rosenfeld, pp. 685-689).

21. **(a)** Immunizations in persons with HIV infection produce an attenuated response with titers being highest in individuals with early HIV or normal or

mildly decreased CD4$^+$ cell counts. In general, live vaccinations are contra-indicated (e.g., live oral polio, bacille Calmette-Guerin (BCG) and yellow fever). MMR is a live vaccine and should be avoided in those with severe immunosuppression. However, because of increased mortality and atypical presentations of measles, those born after 1956 without documented vaccination or history of measles should receive MMR. The Centers for Disease Control and Prevention recommends the pneumococcal vaccine, *Haemophilus influenzae*, influenza vaccine, and hepatitis B vaccine if titers are negative (Fihn & DeWitt, pp. 686-687).

22. **(c)** All systems can be effected by the HIV virus, but the most serious complications are seen in the pulmonary, gastrointestinal, and neurologic systems. Many conditions are exacerbated by HIV infection, and other infections are relatively unique to HIV positive individuals such as Kaposi's sarcoma and benign parotid lymphoepithelial lesions. Pulmonary infections of HIV are extremely common. Swallowing disorders are common in AIDS patients and may occur during primary HIV infection. In late HIV infection, neurologic complications become increasingly common with atypical and overlapping presentations frequently seen (Fihn & DeWitt, pp. 704-709).

References

Fihn, S., & DeWitt, D. (1998). *Outpatient medicine*. Philadelphia, W. B. Saunders.

Rosenfeld, J. (1997). *Women's health in primary care*. Baltimore: Williams & Wilkins.

Tierney, Jr., L. M., McPhee, S. J., & Padadakis, M. A. (1998). *Current medical diagnosis and treatment* (37th ed.). Stamford, CT: Appleton & Lange.

Pregnancy, Contraception and Menopause

Carol Gemberling

Select one best answer to the following questions.

1. The appearance of cervical mucus during ovulation and peak fertility is best described as:

    a. Low volume, cloudy, thick and low elasticity
    b. High volume, clear, thin, and high elasticity
    c. Low volume, cloudy, ferning and minimum cellularity
    d. High volume, thin, clear, and no ferning

2. Which of the following statements best describes the benefits of using condoms instead of other readily available contraceptive methods?

    a. Condom use requires male cooperation and involvement, which encourages their involement in contraception
    b. Condoms have been shown to increase sensitivity and enhance erection in most of the men who use them regularly
    c. Condoms provide for sexually transmitted infection protection and can be used with other contraceptive methods
    d. Allergies to latex condoms, spermacidal agents, and condom breakage are extremely rare

3. Which of the following statements best describes the noncontraceptive benefits of taking combination oral contraceptives for a normal healthy, nonpregnant woman in a mutually monogamous relationship?

    a. The incidence of chlamydia infections and cervical ectopy is decreased among oral contraceptive pill users
    b. The incidence of gallbladder disease and benign liver tumors is decreased in oral contraceptive pill users

c. The incidence of ovarian and endometrial cancer is decreased in oral contraceptive pill users

d. The incidence of thrombophlebitis and pulmonary emboli are decreased in oral contraceptive pill users

4. Which one of the following statements represents the best reason to consider a progestin only pill over a combination oral contraceptive pill?

a. It provides more contraceptive effectiveness than combination pills when taken correctly

b. It has a lower incidence of irregular bleeding than combination pills when taken correctly

c. It can be taken by women who have had breast tenderness with combination pills

d. It can be taken by women who experienced hypertension on combination pills

5. Which of the following statements is correct regarding the use of medroxy-progesterone injections as a contraceptive method?

a. Satisfaction with this method may increase if clients are told to anticipate menstrual cycle irregularity during the first year with increasing likelihood of amenorrhea in subsequent years

b. Satisfaction with this method is increased when women are attempting to lose weight because this method provides less weight gain than other hormonal contraceptive agents

c. Future fertility is readily reversible after the three month interval of effectiveness and may therefore be a good method for this client

d. This method is an excellent choice for women with irregular menses, increased days of light bleeding, spotting, or amenorrhea because of the stabilizing effect on the endometrium

6. Ms. Lewis is a 30-year-old divorced woman who would like to use an IUD as her contraceptive method since she used one very successfully while married. She has two school-age children and is currently dating a man who has never had children. She wants a highly effective method because she is happy with the size of her family, but can't decide if a more permanent method is right for her at this time. Which of the following statements best reflects a consideration regarding the selection of an IUD as a method of choice?

a. Women who have had children demonstrate a decreased incidence of pelvic inflammatory disease when using an IUD for contraception

   b. Women who have contraindications to hormonal methods of contraception can use an IUD

   c. Women who use an IUD for contraception have a decreased incidence of ectopic pregnancy than women using other contraceptive methods

   d. Women who choose an IUD for contraception can have it inserted at any time in their menstrual cycle regardless of present contraceptive history

7. Which of the following statements is true regarding vasectomy and female sterilization?

   a. Vasectomy is simpler, safer, and less expensive than female surgical contraception

   b. Female surgical contraception is more effective, less painful, and more quickly performed than vasectomy

   c. Female surgical contraception has fewer postoperative problems as compared to vasectomy

   d. Reversal of either procedure is safe, inexpensive, and return to fertility is likely

8. While waiting for the vasectomy to be performed, Ms. Lewis and Mr. Johns have a single act of midcycle unprotected intercourse. Apparently the condom they were using last night broke and they are now concerned that pregnancy may take place. What is the best response to this dilemma?

   a. Emergency contraception is inappropriate as risk of conceiving is less than 5%

   b. Emergency contraception is available within 72 hours of unprotected sex

   c. Postcoital insertion of an IUD would be an appropriate selection in this case and they should be scheduled to come back next week for the procedure

   d. They should wait until her period is due and come into the office if it is delayed or abnormal

9. The diaphragm, when used with contraceptive jelly, has not been shown to reduce the:

   a. Incidence of HIV in women who use the diaphragm regularly

   b. Risk of chlamydia and gonorrhea in women who use the diaphragm regularly

   c. Risk of PID and ectopic pregnancy in women who use the diaphragm regularly

   d. Risk of cervical neoplasia in women who use the diaphragm regularly

10. The cervical cap offers contraceptive benefits to women who are not good candidates for the diaphragm. Which of the following statements best describes the women who would benefit from the cervical cap instead of the diaphragm?

    a. Women with a history of toxic shock syndrome are better candidates for the cap rather than the diaphragm

    b. Women with an abnormal Pap smear tolerate a cervical cap better than a diaphragm

    c. Women seen at the first postpartum or postabortion visit are good candidates for the cervical cap instead of the diaphragm

    d. Women who have multiple acts of intercourse over a one to two day period may find the cap easier to use than the diaphragm

11. Which of the following statements best describes the physiology of ovulation?

    a. Normally the corpus luteum life span is variable and may continue to be functional for up to three weeks

    b. Ovulation takes place 12 to 16 days before the onset of menstruation and is therefore not a reliable indication of fertility

    c. Progesterone secretion is predominate in the first half of the menstrual cycle and stimulates the FSH and LH surge at midcycle

    d. Ovulation takes place two weeks after menstruation starts and is a reliable indicator of fertility

Questions 12, 13, 14, and 15 refer to the following scenario.

Mr. and Mrs. Gutierrez, both in good health and in their early thirties, present for an infertility evaluation. They have been attempting to conceive their first child for over one year. Their histories are negative for any sexually transmitted infections, endocrine abnormalities, or congenital, gynecologic, or urologic conditions. They deny any known exposures or lifestyle factors which could contribute to a low sperm count. Foam and condoms have been used in the past. Despite a history of regular 28 to 30 day cycles with intercourse every other day, conception has not occurred.

12. Which of the following best describes the sequence in which an infertility evaluation would proceed after a complete male and female history and physical examination?

    a. Semen evaluation, begin ovulatory indicators, then postcoital test

    b. Serum progesterone level, thyroid panel, then endometrial biopsy

    c. Postcoital test, hysterosalpingogram, then testosterone level

    d. Male and female hormone evaluation, sperm immunologic studies, then diagnostic laparoscopy

13. Mr. and Mrs. Gutierrez were able to conceive within two months without the use of any infertility therapies. As part of your first prenatal pelvic examination you find signs which are associated with early pregnancy. Which of the following statements best describes anticipated normal findings 11 weeks after the last menstrual period?

    a. Uterine fundal height half way between the symphysis pubis and the umbilicus, positive fetal movement, and fetal heart tones of 160 beats per minute with the fetoscope

    b. Lower uterine segment softening and asymmetry of the uterine body, fetal heart tones at 140 beats per minute with the doppler, and nausea

    c. Uterine fundus palpable just below the symphysis pubis, linea nigra, spontaneous colostrum, and Braxton-Hicks contractions

    d. Globular, spongy, tender uterine body palpable 2 cm above the symphysis pubis, bluish discoloration of the vulvovaginal area, and no audible heart tones with the doppler

14. Mrs. Gutierrez reports that she doesn't like to take pills unless absolutely necessary. She is willing to do anything you suggest to ensure a normal pregnancy and a healthy baby. She asks you what the clinic's policy is regarding vitamins and other supplements in pregnancy. Which of the following statements best reflects current thinking with regards to supplementation of vitamins and minerals in pregnancy?

    a. Multivitamins supplemented with iron, folic acid, and calcium routinely given to pregnant woman clearly demonstrate improved pregnancy outcomes.

    b. Folic acid supplementation taken preconceptually and in early pregnancy has been shown to reduce the incidence of neural tube defects

    c. Iron supplementation has been shown to improve pregnancy outcomes with regards to the incidence of preterm deliveries, low birth weight and neonatal deaths

    d. Multivitamins should routinely be taken by vegetarians because their diet is generally low in complete proteins, vitamin D, and calcium

15. Mrs. Gutierrez is now in her second trimester and reports that she has been experiencing painless vaginal bleeding for the last two days and doesn't know

what may be causing the bleeding. She and her husband stopped having inter-course two weeks ago and she has been taking it easy since she stopped work-ing last week. Her baby's activity continues to be the same as it has been over the past few weeks. What is the next step in the management of this patient?

a. An ultrasound should be done to detect a low lying placenta
b. A digital vaginal examination should be done to assess for cervical soft-ening
c. A nonstress test should be performed to assess fetal viability
d. A kick count should be initiated to assess fetal well being

16. Ms. Wilcox is an 18-year-old woman gravida 2 para 1 who presents for the first time for prenatal care. Her last menstrual period was approximately 28 weeks ago and since her first baby was born "early" she believes that the con-tractions she began feeling last evening are true labor. Which of the following is not a factor in the development of preterm labor?

a. Increased maternal age with the second or third birth, overhydration, sed-entary employment, and uterine contractions of 1 to 2 per hour
b. Maternal age less than 18, previous preterm birth, maternal genitourinary tract infection with chlamydia, or asymptomatic bacteriuria
c. Maternal psychosocial stress, work involving heavy lifting, cigarette and other substance abuse, or inappropriate working conditions
d. Greater than 4 to 6 uterine contraction per hour, uterine anomalies, and conditions that abnormally distend the uterus

17. During a two week postpartum examination your patient complains of flu-like symptoms and a red tender area on her breast. Which of the following state-ments best describes the organism most frequently isolated in mastitis and its usual route of transmission?

a. *Enterobacter cloacae* is frequently transmitted to the breast via the oral-fe-cal route
b. β-*hemolytic streptococcus* is frequently transmitted via a hematogenous spread
c. *Pseudomonas aeruginosa* is frequently transmitted from hospital personnel
d. *Staphylococcus aureus* is frequently transmitted through an irritated or cracked nipple

18. Mrs. Williams is a 58-year-old thin, relaxed, postmenopausal woman who pres-ents for a well-woman examination. While performing the bimanual examina-tion, you palpate a 3 by 3 cm round, well defined mass just lateral to the right uterine fundus. What is the appropriate response to this finding?

   a. Tell the patient that this is an expected finding in a woman of her age

   b. Tell the patient that this is probably stool and that follow up is unnecessary

   c. Have her perform three fecal occult blood tests and refer her for a sigmoidoscopy

   d. Order pelvic ultrasound, CA_{125}, and schedule referral to gynecologist

19. While performing a well-woman examination on a postmenopausal woman who is not taking hormone replacement therapy, you would expect to see changes associated with the cessation of endogenous female hormone production. Which of the following would not be an expected finding in a postmenopausal woman?

   a. Vaginal dryness, insertional dyspareunia, vulvar burning and urinary symptoms

   b. Forgetfulness, insomnia, difficulty concentrating, mood lability, and depression

   c. Urinary frequency, vaginal spotting, and dyspareunia with deep penetration

   d. Hot flashes, night sweats, fluid retention, myalgias, and tiredness

20. Various hormone replacement therapy regimens are available to postmenopausal women who have no contraindications to estrogen either alone or in combination with progestin. Which of the following statements is inaccurate with regard to hormone replacement therapy?

   a. Estrogen and progestin therapy are indicated for a woman who has had a hysterectomy

   b. Estrogen therapy alone can be taken daily by a woman who has had a hysterectomy

   c. Progestin can be added every three to four months to estrogen taken 25 days of the month

   d. Estrogen dose equivalent to 0.625 mg is adequate to prevent osteoporosis in 90% of women

21. Women considering hormone replacement therapy need to be made aware of potential risks and benefits of therapeutic options. Which of the following statements best describes the current thinking regarding the risk benefit analysis of long term estrogen therapy for healthy postmenopausal women with positive health behaviors?

   a. The lifetime risk of developing endometrial and breast cancer is three times greater than the risk of developing and dying from coronary artery disease

b. The lifetime risk of developing coronary artery disease is nearly twice as great as the probability of developing endometrial and breast cancer combined

c. The lifetime probability of a Caucasian woman developing breast cancer is greater than her probability of developing osteoporosis

d. The lifetime probability of a woman developing cardiovascular disease is greater than the combined risk of her developing osteoporosis, breast, or endometrial cancer combined

22. Atrophic vaginitis is a common problem in postmenopausal women. Which of the following management plans is most appropriate for women with this troubling condition?

a. Treatment with topical vaginal antibiotics will usually clear up atrophic vaginitis

b. Vaginal moisturizers make intercourse more comfortable and stimulate natural secretions

c. Acidifying the vaginal pH to 4 will eliminate the long term problem with lactobacilli

d. Treatment with topical estrogen can be used even if contraindications to oral therapy exist

Answers and Rationale

1. **(b)** Midcycle cervical mucus is likely to be high volume, thin, clear, and ferning, with minimum cellularity and high elasticity (Hatcher, et al., p. 72).

2. **(c)** Many male patients will not use condoms because of the issues of sensitivity, interference with erection, decreased pleasure, and male involvement for birth control. Latex and spermicidal allergic reactions are seen fairly often in clinical practice and breakage, although rare, is still seen as a potential problem with the use of condoms. Latex condoms have been shown to be the best contraceptive agent that can potentially protect against sexually transmitted infections and pregnancy. Abstinence is the only 100% effective method to prevent both pregnancy and infection (Hatcher, et al., pp. 325-355).

3. **(c)** A decreased incidence of ovarian and endometrial cancer is known to be one of the leading noncontraceptive benefits to taking oral contraceptives. The remaining choices all represent known risks to individuals who take oral contraceptives (Hatcher, et al., pp. 409-410).

4. **(d)** Progestin pills have a lower efficacy rate, produce more irregular bleeding, and are generally taken by women considering levonorgestrel implants or medroxyprogesterone injections before these methods are initiated to see if progestin is tolerated by the client. The progestin only "minipill" is frequently used by women who can not tolerate or have contraindications for estrogen containing contraception. Women who are breastfeeding and desire oral contraception are good candidates for the progestin only "minipill" (Hatcher, et al., pp. 429-434).

5. **(a)** Medroxyprogesterone injections are not a good contraceptive choice in women who may want a prompt return of fertility, have a concern about weight gain, or have had unexplained abnormal vaginal bleeding within the past three months. Method satisfaction is greater if the impact of bleeding changes is understood, and if women are informed in advance (Hatcher, et al., pp. 473-487).

6. **(b)** The careful selection of candidates for IUD insertion can make a difference in effectiveness and safety. IUD use increases the risk of PID, with the greatest risk at the time of insertion. If a woman should become pregnant

while using an IUD, the chance of that pregnancy being ectopic is greater than it would be with other contraceptive methods. Women with a questionable or unknown history of reliable contraception used in the most recent menstrural cycle should not have an IUD inserted until pregnancy can be ruled out. However, a copper IUD is a good contraceptive choice for women who cannot tolerate, or have contraindications to, hormonal methods (Hatcher, et al., pp. 515-522).

7. **(a)** Male and female sterilization should be considered permanent methods of contraception because reversal is expensive, requires major surgery and special surgical skills, and success is not guaranteed. Vasectomy continues to be the safest and most cost effective contraceptive method for men and women. Female sterilization is a more technically difficult procedure than vasectomy and carries a higher morbidity and mortality than vasectomy (Hatcher, et al., pp. 548-552).

8. **(b)** Emergency contraception is one of the most under utilized methods available to sexually active couples. Because a vasectomy is their method of choice, oral contraceptive postcoital contraception is superior to IUD insertion, with its inherent risks of insertion and cost. The risk of pregnancy with one act of midcycle unprotected intercourse ranges from approximately 15% to 26%. Accidents can happen with even the most reliable couples, and no assumptions should be drawn about contraceptive desires and wishes with a single act of contraceptive method failure. Waiting until menstruation is delayed will only complicate the choices and actions that may be taken in this case (Hatcher, et al., pp. 280-290).

9. **(a)** The impact of vaginal barriers on HIV risk is not known. Chlamydia, gonorrhea, PID, ectopic pregnancies, and cervical neoplasia risk reduction have all been documented in women who are regular users of the diaphragm, spermicides or male condoms (Hatcher, et al., pp. 379-382).

10. **(d)** Many similarities exist between the diaphragm and cervical cap. Contraindications for both methods include a past history of toxic shock syndrome or known or suspected cervical neoplasia. Immediate postpartum and post-abortion fitting is not desirable as accurate fitting can not occur until full involution is obtained. The cervical cap may be easier to use when a woman has multiple acts of intercourse over a 1 or 2 day time period (Hatcher, et al., p. 378).

11. **(b)** The follicular or preovulatory phase of the menstrual cycle is somewhat variable and can not be used as a reliable indicator of when ovulation will take place. The luteal postovulatory phase is 14 days with a two day variability in either direction. This makes the date of the menstrual period a helpful sign of ovulation but only retrospectively. Young women frequently have a year or so of anovulatory cycles in which bleeding occurs in irregular cycles and is not associated with fertility. Estrogen dominates in the first half of the menstrual cycle and impacts the FSH and LH surge seen just prior to ovulation (Hatcher, et al., pp. 70-74).

12. **(a)** The initial assessment of couples should proceed in a systematic manner, with the objective of completing the first line of infertility evaluation within approximately 2 to 3 cycles. After a complete and infertility focused history and physical examination is performed on both partners, the next most appropriate test is the semen analysis. Male and female blood tests may be performed but are frequently delayed until later in the infertility evaluation in normal couples. Ovulatory indicators include tracking the basal body temperature, fertility awareness record keeping, or other reliable and readily available ovulation detection kits. The evaluation proceeds from least invasive and costly to most invasive and costly, with the postcoital test, serum progesterone, and other blood tests being sequenced next. Endometrial biopsy, hysterosalpingogram, and other diagnostic studies such as laparoscopy, hormone studies, and immunologic studies may be performed depending on the above findings (Hatcher, et al., pp. 665-670).

13. **(b)** The uterine body at 11 weeks will begin to be a palpable abdominal structure just behind the symphysis pubis in lean women. Fetal heart tones should be heard in most women by 11 weeks since the last period, and softening of the lower uterine segment (Hegar's sign) and asymmetry of the uterine body (Piskacek's sign) can be palpated. Fetal heart tones should be approximately 120 to 160 beats per minute and nausea may still be present at 11 menstrual weeks. The linea nigra usually doesn't appear until much later in pregnancy and the appearance of colostrum is usually seen in the second trimester. Braxton Hicks contractions are more likely to be felt in the third trimester in most women but may need evaluation and monitoring if experienced earlier in pregnancy (Ratcliff, et al., pp. 15-16, 35, 43-47, 88-90).

14. **(b)** Multivitamins have traditionally been given to healthy pregnant women despite the absence of disease with no improvement in pregnancy outcomes

seen in retrospective clinical trials. Except for supplementation with folic acid, no improvement in pregnancy outcomes has been shown as a result of the use of these preparations. Routine iron supplementation has not been shown in retrospective clinical trials to improve pregnancy outcomes. Vitamins can not replace protein deficiencies that might be seen in strict vegetarians (Ratcliff, et al., pp. 54-55).

15. **(a)** An ultrasound is the best next step for Mrs. Gutierez. A digital examination in a pregnant woman who is experiencing vaginal bleeding could be catastrophic if the cervix is dilated and the placenta is over the cervical os. A carefully performed, sterile speculum examination, or vaginal ultrasound evaluation of the lower uterine segment, may be helpful in making the diagnosis of placenta previa. A nonstress test and a kick count may be helpful indicators of fetal well being and activity, but are not the best first step in this case (Ratcliff, et al., pp. 117-118, 329-330, 361-362).

16. **(a)** All of the factors listed play a role in or have an association with the development of preterm labor except for overhydration, sedentary employment, and infrequent uterine contraction. Advanced maternal age is a factor in the development of preterm labor especially with first deliveries (Ratcliff, et al., pp. 219-223).

17. **(d)** Even though the other organisms are infrequently isolated as a cause of acute mastitis, the organism is thought to gain access through a cracked or irritated nipple (Ratcliff, et al., pp. 439-440).

18. **(d)** A postmenopausal woman's uterus and ovaries should involute in the postmenopausal period. Any well defined adnexal mass warrants further diagnostic evaluation (Ratcliff, et al., p. 481; Barkaukas, et al., p. 555).

19. **(c)** All of the symptoms listed may be experienced in a postmenopausal woman except urinary frequency, vaginal spotting, and deep dyspareunia which may be signs of pathologic conditions needing further investigation and diagnosis (Rosenfeld, pp. 788-793).

20. **(a)** Many therapeutic regimes exist for women wishing to take hormone replacement. Progestin therapy need not be taken along with estrogen

replacement in a woman who has had a hysterectomy because there is no endometrium to protect (Rosenfeld, pp. 776-781).

21. **(d)** Utilizing lifetime risk statistics is one way to look at the risk benefit analysis of taking exogenous hormone therapy. Although there is disagreement in the risk benefit estimates, the following figures represent consensus from the literature: Lifetime risk of endometrial cancer 2.6%, breast cancer 10%, osteoporosis 15%, lifetime probability for Caucasian women developing osteoporosis 10% to 20%; lifetime probability of developing coronary artery disease 46%, with 31% dying from coronary heart disease (Rosenfeld, pp. 763-771).

22. **(b)** Atrophic vaginitis is a common vaginal disorder seen in women not taking estrogen. It is caused by a change of predominant bacterial species from lactobacilli dominant normal flora to a dominant coliform type of bacterial flora. In addition, a change in the vaginal pH from approximately 4 to a level of 6.5 to 7, and a thinning of the vaginal mucosa, increases the risk of infections. Estrogen is the specific drug of choice to treat and prevent atrophic vaginitis. Vaginal lubricants can be used alone or until estrogen topical creams restore the vaginal mucosa. Vaginal moisturizers last up to 72 hours and help stimulate natural secretions (Rosenfeld, pp. 499-500, 776).

References

Barkaukas, V., & Stoltenberg-Allen, K., & Baumann, L. C., & Darling-Fisher, C. D. (1998). *Health and physical assessment*. St. Louis: Mosby.

Hatcher, R. A., Trussel, J., Stewart, F., Cates, W., Stewart, G. K., Guest, F., & Kowal, D. (1998). *Contraceptive technology* (17th ed.). NY: Ardent Media.

Ratcliff, S., Byrd, J., & Sakornbut, E. (1996). *Handbook of pregnancy and perinatal care in family practice: Science and practice*. Philadelphia: Hanley & Belfus.

Rosenfeld, J. (1997). *Women's health in primary care*. Baltimore: Williams & Wilkins.

Musculoskeletal Disorders

Cheryl Ahern-Lehmann

Select one best answer to the following questions.

Questions 1, 2, and 3 refer to the following scenario.

Jay Green, a 45-year-old male, presents with a chief complaint of low back pain which began after shoveling snow from his driveway two weeks ago. He reports intermittent burning pain down the back of his left leg to his ankle. He denies any recent or past history of back trauma.

1. To rule out an emergent cauda equina syndrome, you would specifically need to ask Mr. Green which of the following questions?

    a. Have you had numbness or tingling down your left leg?
    b. Have you had urinary retention or incontinence?
    c. Have you had any pain in your groin or perineum?
    d. Has coughing or sneezing intensified your pain?

2. During Mr. Green's physical examination you note left ankle dorsiflexion weakness and left great toe extensor weakness to resistance. These weaknesses suggest a possible disk herniation in which intervertebral space?

    a. L_3 to L_4
    b. L_4 to L_5
    c. L_5 to S_1
    d. S_1 to S_2

3. Which of the following interventions would not be recommended in the initial two weeks of treatment for Mr. Green's acute low back pain?

    a. An elastic back corset
    b. Back massage
    c. Low stress aerobic stretching exercise
    d. Muscle relaxants

4. Which of the following types of arthritis is HLA-B27 positive?

   a. Osteoarthritis
   b. Gonococcal arthritis
   c. Rheumatoid arthritis
   d. Ankylosing spondylitis

5. Which of the following radiographic joint changes might you expect to see in rheumatoid arthritis?

   a. Narrowing of joint spaces and osteophyte formation
   b. Erosion and sclerosis of the sacroiliac joints
   c. Soft tissue swelling, osteoporosis, and joint narrowing
   d. Punched out areas of bone adjacent to soft tissue lesions

6. Which of the following drugs is usually the first employed in the early treatment of rheumatoid arthritis?

   a. Ibuprofen
   b. Methotrexate
   c. Corticosteroids
   d. Gold salts

7. Amy Graham, a 22-year-old female college student, limps into the clinic with pain in her left knee. She tells you that last night, while playing basketball, she pivoted quickly and experienced severe pain in her knee which forced her to stop playing. Since then the knee has slowly become increasingly swollen, painful with full weight-bearing, and she has experienced an intermittent "catching" sensation. On examination you find that she has a left knee joint effusion, medial joint line tenderness, is unable to deep knee bend or duck walk, and has a positive McMurray's sign. This history and physical findings suggest that Amy may have a(n):

   a. Medial meniscus tear
   b. Medial collateral ligament tear
   c. Anterior cruciate ligament tear
   d. Posterior cruciate ligament tear

8. Which of the following is the most sensitive test for systemic lupus erythematosus?

   a. LE cell preparation
   b. Antinuclear antibody
   c. Erythrocyte sedimentation rate

d. Anti-native DNA

Questions 9, 10, and 11 refer to the following scenario.

Brad Berry, a 36-year-old male, presents to your office with a red, "hot," swollen, painful right knee. He first noticed the problem last night, and feels it has gotten worse over the last 14 hours.

9. In your immediate considerations of differential diagnoses for Mr. Berry's knee problem, which of the following would be least likely?

    a. Trauma
    b. Septic arthritis
    c. Rheumatoid arthritis
    d. Acute gout

Your medical history reveals that Mr. Berry denies problems with any other joints or recent injury to his right knee. He is sexually active, monogamous for three years, and denies urethral discharge or urinary symptoms, recent rash, IV drug use, or chronic illness. His temperature is 102.2° F.

10. With this information, what is the most likely diagnosis for Mr. Berry's knee problem?

    a. Gonococcal arthritis
    b. Acute gout
    c. Lyme disease
    d. Rheumatoid arthritis

11. Which of the following would be the most definitive test for determining the true diagnosis of Mr. Berry's knee problem?

    a. Right knee joint radiograph
    b. Right knee joint synovial fluid examination
    c. Serum rheumatoid factor
    d. Serum erythrocyte sedimentation rate

12. A positive Finkelstein test suggests which of the following pathologies?

    a. de Quervain's synotendinitis
    b. Carpal tunnel syndrome
    c. Ulnar tunnel syndrome
    d. Dupuytren's contracture

Questions 13 and 14 refer to the following scenario.

Emma Lang, a 62-year-old female, comes into your office two hours after being in an automobile accident in which she sustained a whiplash injury to her neck.

13. If Mrs. Lang told you that she had immediate pain in the back of her neck and head after the accident, and that the pain has been constant since then, what problem is it critical to rule out immediately?

    a. Torticollis
    b. Cervical spine fracture
    c. Cervical disk herniation
    d. Concussion

14. Upon history, Mrs. Lang denies loss of consciousness, dizziness, visual disturbances, nausea, vomiting, and arm paresthesias or weakness. Her musculoskeletal examination is unremarkable except for generalized tenderness in the anterior and posterior neck musculature. Her neurological examination is negative for pathology, and her cervical spine radiograph is negative. Which of the treatment regimens below would initially be best for Mrs. Lang?

    a. Ice frequently for 48 hours, begin muscle relaxants, and start physical therapy
    b. Alternate ice and wet heat frequently for 48 hours, begin NSAID and physical therapy
    c. Wet heat frequently for 48 hours, begin muscle relaxants, soft cervical collar for two weeks
    d. Ice frequently for 48 hours, rest, soft cervical collar for 1 to 2 days, begin NSAID

15. Which of the following dermatome patterns is typical of the pain and/or paresthesia distribution resulting from C_6 cervical nerve root compression?

    a. Volar and dorsal aspects of the radial side of the forearm, wrist, and hand, including the thumb and first finger
    b. Volar and dorsal aspects of the ulnar side of the forearm, wrist, and hand, including the 4th and 5th fingers
    c. The palmar and dorsal aspects of the hand, including the third finger
    d. The volar and dorsal aspects of the medial forearm and elbow

16. Which of the following patterns of low back pain would increase your suspicion of the possibility of malignancy?

    a. Pain aggravated by activity and alleviated by rest

b. Acute, writhing pain
c. Pain that improves with activity and worsens with rest
d. Pain at night, unrelieved by rest or the supine position

17. A 25-year-old male comes in to your office complaining of a sore right wrist and hand. The patient tells you that he tripped three days ago, fell forward, and "caught" himself by landing on his outstretched hands. Since then he has had increasing pain and swelling in his right wrist. Upon examination you note right wrist swelling and tenderness, without redness or ecchymosis. The wrist joint is stable, with only slightly limited range of motion, and the patient has a very tender "snuffbox." These findings suggest which of the following injuries?

   a. Fracture of the radial head
   b. Scaphoid/navicular fracture
   c. Sprain of wrist ligaments
   d. Dislocation of the distal ulna

18. A 42-year-old male comes in for evaluation of pain in his right elbow. He tells you that he has intermittent numbness and tingling from his elbow to his lateral forearm and hand. He feels that his dominant right forearm has become "weak" and that worries him because he is a garbage collector and needs to lift heavy trash barrels every day. Upon examination you find that he has increased pain on flexion of his right elbow, and a positive Tinel's sign behind the medial epicondyle which "sends a tingling, like an electrical current" into the lateral side of his right hand, including the 4th and 5th fingers. The diagnosis for his elbow problem is most likely:

   a. Epicondylitis/tennis elbow
   b. Degenerative joint disease of the elbow
   c. Olecranon bursitis
   d. Cubital tunnel syndrome

19. Which of the following medications has been demonstrated to have modest efficacy, and is now commonly recommended for the treatment of the pain of fibromyalgia (fibrositis)?

   a. Naproxen
   b. Hydrocodone with acetaminophen
   c. Amitriptyline
   d. Prednisone

20. The initial treatment for plantar fasciitis is usually:

a. Heel pad, NSAID, and exercises to stretch plantar fascia
b. Cortisone injection and exercises to stretch plantar fascia
c. Heel pad, cortisone injection, and hot and cold soaks
d. Hot and cold soaks, heel pad, and exercises to stretch plantar fascia

21. Initial pharmacologic treatment for an acute episode of gouty arthritis would include:

a. Indomethacin or allopurinol
b. Aspirin or colchicine
c. Indomethacin or colchicine
d. Aspirin or probenecid

22. Most cases of Reiter's syndrome (reactive arthritis) are thought to develop within days or weeks of an episode of which of the following diseases?

a. Salmonella dysentery
b. Inflammatory bowel disease
c. Psoriasis
d. Gonorrhea

Answers and Rationale

1. **(b)** Cauda equina syndrome can be ruled out with a medical history that ascertains the absence of bladder dysfunction (usually urinary retention or overflow incontinence), saddle anesthesia, and unilateral or bilateral leg pain and weakness. Bowel incontinence and impotence can also be indicators of a cauda equina process (USDHHS, p. 16; Mercier, p. 141; Goroll, et al., p. 745; Tierney, et al., p. 785).

2. **(b)** A herniated disk at L_4 to L_5 is documented in 80% of patients with ankle dorsiflexion weakness and 30% of patients with great toe extensor weakness (USDHHS, pp. 18-19; Mercier, p. 141; Tierney, et al., p. 786.; Weinstock & Neides, p. 170).

3. **(a)** The AHCPR panel on acute low back pain states "lumbar corsets and support belts have not been proven beneficial for treating patients with acute low back problems." Other sources question the value of corsets or traction. All other treatments listed are recommended for the initial treatment of acute low back pain (USDHHS, p. 39; Tierney, et al., pp. 786–787; Weinstock & Neides, p. 171).

4. **(d)** HLA-B27 is positive in 90% of patients with ankylosing spondylitis. Osteoarthritis, rheumatoid arthritis, and gonococcal arthritis are usually HLA-B27 negative (Tierney, et al., p. 811).

5. **(c)** Radiologic changes in rheumatoid arthritis include osteoporosis, severe joint space narrowing, joint erosion, and soft-tissue swelling. Radiologic changes listed in "a" are those typical of osteoarthritis. Radiologic changes listed in "b" are those of ankylosing spondylitis; those listed in "d" are radiologic findings consistent with chronic gout (Mercier, p. 285; Tierney, et al., p. 711; Wells, et al., p. 29).

6. **(a)** NSAIDs are the first line drugs of choice for initial treatment of rheumatoid arthritis unless their use is contraindicated. They act as both analgesics and anti-inflammatories, as they block the synthesis of prostaglandins involved in the inflammatory cascade (Tierney, et al., p. 793; Wells, et al., pp. 31–32).

7. **(a)** Meniscal injuries often occur with a twisting force applied to the knee with the extremity bearing weight, are often associated with sudden pain, gradual swelling, joint line tenderness, locking or catching, inability to duck walk, and a positive McMurray's sign (Mercier p. 318; Bergfeld, et al., pp. 103, 108).

8. **(b)** Antinuclear antibody tests are the most sensitive (but not specific) tests for systemic lupus erythematosus; 95% to 100% of lupus patients have a positive serum ANA (Goroll, et al., p. 741; Tierney, et al., p. 799).

9. **(c)** Rheumatoid arthritis is classically a polyarticular joint disease, which usually presents in the metacarpal phalangeal and wrist joints; it also predominantly occurs in women. Gout, trauma, septic arthritis, and Lyme disease are more apt to present as acute monarticular problems in the knee, as in this patient (Tierney, et al., p. 775; Mercier, p. 282; Goroll, et al., pp. 732–733).

10. **(b)** Gout can occur acutely (often at night), is monarticular, and occurs often in the knee. Fever is a common associated finding, as with Mr. Berry. Gonococcal arthritis more commonly has a septic course with a prodrome of migratory polyarthralgias and skin rash, is more common in women, and less than 50% of patients have fever. Lyme disease is a more systemic disease, usually with erythema migrans, flu-like symptoms, fever, chills, myalgia, and headache or stiff neck. Lyme arthritis can be monarticular, but is usually more chronic and recurrent. Rheumatoid arthritis is classically a polyarticular disease of the smaller joints, and occurs more often in women. Prodromal systemic symptoms of malaise, fever, and weight loss are associated with rheumatoid arthritis (Tierney, et al., pp. 775, 778, 791, 1318-1319; Mercier, pp. 278-293; Wells, et al., p. 3).

11. **(b)** Joint fluid aspiration and analysis would be the most definitive test listed for sudden, onset, "hot" monarticular joint disease. Synovial fluid analysis would identify uric acid crystals in gout and elevated leukocytes and bacteria in bacterial infections/septic joints. Knee radiograph is commonly negative in early gout, early rheumatoid arthritis, gonococcal arthritis, or Lyme disease. Neither the rheumatoid factor, nor the ESR are definitive of, or specific for, diagnosis of monarticular acute joint disease (Tierney, et al., pp. 775–776, 778, 791, 1318-1319; Mercier, p. 282; Goroll, et al., pp. 733, 741; Wells, et al., p. 3).

12. **(a)** The Finklestein test reproduces the pain of de Quervain's tenosynovitis by passively flexing the thumb and adducting the wrist, and stretching the extensor pollicis brevis and abductor pollicis longus over the radial styloid (Goroll, et al., p. 771; Mercier, p. 106).

13. **(b)** The usual pain and stiffness associated with whiplash injury comes on gradually, hours after the injury occurred. If neck pain was immediate at the time of the injury and continues uninterrupted, "the injury should be treated as a cervical spine fracture until proven otherwise" (Pearson, p. 14).

14. **(d)** Initial treatment of whiplash injuries includes rest, traction (a soft cervical collar for a limited time; recommendations vary from 1 to 2 days to two weeks), anti-inflammatories (NSAID), and ice for the first 48 hours. Heat is avoided during the first 48 hours, but used later. ROM exercises/physical therapy are usually begun only after the initial acute pain is over. Muscle relaxants are controversial, but can be used for significant muscle spasm and discomfort; they are usually started later, if at all (Goroll, et al., p. 753; Mercier, pp. 39-40; Pearson, pp. 17-20; Tierney, et al., p. 782).

15. **(a)** Answer choice "a" describes the C_6 dermatome pattern in the forearm and hand (Mercier, p. 33; Tierney, et al., p. 966).

16. **(d)** Approximately 90% of patients with spinal neoplasms report night pain unrelieved by lying down (supine position) or bed rest. The patterns of pain described in the other answer choices are not typical of malignancy (Goroll, et al., p. 744; Tierney, et al., p. 704).

17. **(b)** Scaphoid and navicular fractures occur as a result of a fall on outstretched hands. Tenderness in the anatomic snuffbox and swelling and pain in the wrist are characteristic findings. It is important not to miss this fracture; it should be treated by short arm cast to facilitate healing because non-union of this fracture and avascular necrosis are risks of this injury (Ethridge, et al., p. 60; Mercier, p. 124).

18. **(d)** Cubital tunnel syndrome consists of painful paresthesias and muscle weakness along the ulnar nerve distribution in the forearm and hand. Tinel's sign is positive behind the medial epicondyle (Mercier, pp. 108-109; Tierney, et al., p. 963).

19. **(c)** "Placebo-controlled trials have demonstrated modest efficacy of amitripty-line, fluoxetine, chlorpromazine, or cyclobenzaprine," but the NSAID is "generally ineffective," and "opioids and corticosteroids are ineffective and should never be used to treat fibrositis (fibromyalgia)" (Tierney, et al., pp. 788-789).

20. **(a)** Initial treatment for plantar fasciitis is listed in option "a" (Dale, et al., p. 161; Goroll, p. 775).

21. **(c)** Indomethacin or colchicine can each be effective in treating the acute symp-toms of gouty arthritis. Some prefer indomethacin (or other NSAID) as first-line treatment, because of the GI toxicity of colchicine, while others use colchicine first, because "75% to 95% of patients with acute gouty ar-thritis respond favorably to colchicine when ingestion of the drug is begun within 12 hours of onset of joint symptoms." Corticosteroids may also be used to treat the symptoms of acute gout, but are usually reserved for pa-tients who cannot take oral NSAID, or for cases resistant to the two other drugs. Low doses of aspirin (< 2 to 3 g/day) inhibit renal excretion of uric acid, aggravating hyperuricemia, and should be avoided by patients with gout. Both probenecid and allopurinol are not used in the treatment of acute gout, but are part of prophylactic regimens to prevent recurrent prob-lems resulting from hyperuricemia (Tierney, et al., p. 779; Wells, et al., pp. 3-6).

22. **(a)** Most cases of Reiter's syndrome (also called "reactive arthritis") occur within days or weeks of either a dysentery-like illness (caused by shigella, salmonella, yersinia, or campylobacter), or a sexually transmitted infection such as *Chlamydia trachomatis* (Tierney, et al., p. 813).

References

Bergfeld, J., Ireland, M. L., & Wojtys, E. M. (1997). Pinpointing the cause of acute knee pain. *Patient Care, 31*(18), 100–117.

Dale, S. J., David, D. J., & Sykes, T. F. (1997). Effective approaches to common foot complaints. *Patient Care, 31*(5), 158–180.

Ethridge, C. P., Maddox, M., & Ruch, D. (1997). Handling common wrist complaints. *Patient Care, 31*(18), 56–75.

Goroll, A. H., May, L. A., & Mulley, A. G. (1995). *Primary care medicine* (3rd ed.). Philadelphia: J. B. Lippincott.

Mercier, L. R. (1995). *Practical orthopedics* (4th ed.). St. Louis: Mosby.

Pearson, J. K. (1995). A prompt response to acute neck pain. *Patient Care, 29*(4), 14–24.

Tierney, Jr., L. M., McPhee, S. J., & Papadakis, M. A. (1998). *Current medical diagnosis and treatment* (37th ed.). Stamford, CT: Appleton & Lange.

U.S. Department of Health and Human Services (USDHHS), Agency for Health Care Policy and Research. (1994). *Clinical practice guideline, Number 14: Acute low back problems in adults.* Washington, DC: Government Printing Office.

Weinstock, M. B., & Neides, D. M. (1996). *The resident's guide to ambulatory care* (2nd ed.). Columbus, OH: Aadem Publishing.

Wells, B. G., DiPiro, J. T., Schwinghammer, T. L., &. Hamilton, C. W. (1998). *Pharmacotherapy handbook.* Stamford, CT: Appleton & Lange.

Neurological Disorders

Cheryl Ahern-Lehmann

Select one best answer to the following questions.

Questions 1 and 2 refer to the following scenario.

Billy James, a 45-year-old man, presents with severe headaches that woke him the last two nights. Each lasted about one hour, then disappeared. He describes a severe, stabbing, burning pain behind his left eye, accompanied by nasal stuffiness and discharge, and tearing from his left eye. The first night he thought the headache could have been caused by several glasses of red wine that he had at a party before he went to bed. Now he is worried, because the headache recurred last night, even though he intentionally avoided alcohol yesterday. He denies any prior history of such headaches, or any family history of headaches.

1. Based only on this information, your initial thought regarding the most likely diagnosis for his headache is:

    a. Migraine headache
    b. Sinusitis
    c. Cluster headache
    d. Cranial mass

2. Which of the following treatments would you recommend to Mr. James if his headache should occur again?

    a. Oral methysergide
    b. Injection of corticosteroid
    c. Inhalation of 100% oxygen
    d. Oral sumatriptan

3. The pain associated with migraine headache is believed to be caused predominantly by which of the following neurovascular mechanisms?

    a. Cerebral edema

b. Cerebral vasodilation

c. Cerebral ischemia

d. Cerebral vasoconstriction

4. Which of the following would most likely trigger or exacerbate a headache?

a. Asparagus, broiled salmon, bright sunlight, plums, rice, hydrochlorothiazide

b. Lima beans, cold shrimp, lack of sleep, roasted nuts, nitroglycerine

c. Corn, fresh baked tuna, loud noise, apples, fruit pie, pasta, propranolol

d. Cabbage, steamed clams, physical exertion, peaches, pasta, acetaminophen

5. Which of the following medications would not commonly be used in prophylactic/preventive treatment of migraine headaches?

a. Amitriptyline

b. Propranolol

c. Sumatriptan

d. Methysergide

Questions 6 and 7 refer to the following scenario.

Reuben Van Doren, a 70-year-old male, presents with a nagging, throbbing left temporal headache of several days duration. He tells you he had some throat pain and jaw stiffness when he tried to eat. He noticed two days ago that his scalp is tender when he combs his hair, and he has some "chills and sweats, off and on." He denies any previous history of headaches, head trauma, or hypertension, but says he "just doesn't feel well the last few days."

6. Given Mr. Van Doren's history, what is your presumptive diagnosis for his headache?

a. Tension headache

b. Prodrome to herpes zoster

c. Temporomandibular joint dysfunction

d. Giant cell arteritis

7. Given Mr. Van Doren's headache presentation and your presumptive diagnosis, it is most important that your history and physical examination document whether or not he has had any changes in:

a. Hearing

b. Vision

   c. Mood
   d. Motor function

8. Paroxysmal lancinating pain that travels from mouth to ear in a middle aged or older patient is commonly associated with which of the following diagnoses?

   a. Bell's palsy
   b. Temporal arteritis
   c. Cluster headache
   d. Trigeminal neuralgia

9. A 65-year-old woman calls you on the telephone to tell you she is frightened because her husband is suddenly having trouble speaking, and couldn't control his right arm and hand enough to get his tooth brush up to his mouth this morning. She tells you that her 70-year-old husband awoke about an hour ago, feeling "a little dizzy," and then his other symptoms began. He is being treated for hypertension with lisinopril and hydrochlorthiazide and had a "mild heart attack" about two years ago, but he has never had "anything like this before." What is the diagnosis for this woman's husband, given the duration of his symptoms?

   a. Stroke
   b. Transient ischemic attack
   c. Hypokalemia
   d. Hypoglycemia

10. Multiple sclerosis is an inflammatory, demyelinating disease, in which MRI studies document plaques and scarring in the:

   a. White matter of the brain and spinal cord
   b. Gray matter of the brain and spinal cord
   c. White and gray matter of the brain
   d. Gray matter of the spinal cord

11. Which of the following are common initial presenting symptoms of multiple sclerosis?

   a. Memory loss, incontinence, emotional lability
   b. Seizure, ataxia, memory loss
   c. Fatigue, weakness in a limb, diplopia
   d. Facial paralysis, personality change, spasticity

12. When you check the voice for hoarseness, observe the uvula to see if it is midline, test the gag reflex, and assess a patient's ability to swallow, you are testing which cranial nerve?

    a. CN VIII
    b. CN IX
    c. CN X *vagus*
    d. CN XI

13. In a patient with Bell's palsy, when you test the corneal reflex in the affected eye, it would be typical to find:

    a. Normal corneal sensation and corneal reflex
    b. Normal corneal sensation, but a decreased corneal reflex √
    c. Decreased corneal sensation, but a normal corneal reflex
    d. Decreased corneal sensation and decreased corneal reflex

14. Which of the following is considered optimal medical management of transient ischemic attacks in patients under age 65?

    a. Aspirin √
    b. Verapamil
    c. Phenytoin
    d. Nitroglycerine

15. Which of the following is a criterion for endarterectomy in patients with TIA?

    a. Recurrent TIA over the last year
    b. High risk of cardiovascular morbidity or mortality
    c. Significant carotid bruit
    d. > 70% carotid stenosis on arteriography

16. A 55-year-old woman has been told that she has chronic carpal tunnel syndrome, with nerve compression, in both wrists. Which of the following signs and symptoms would not be consistent with that diagnosis?

    a. Numbness, tingling, and pain in the palmar surface and several fingers of the hand at night
    b. Tapping the volar aspect of the wrist causes paresthesias in the fourth and fifth fingers
    c. Paresthesias into the palm and fingers after 30 to 60 seconds of sustained passive wrist flexion (90 degrees)
    d. Bilateral atrophy of the thenar muscles

17. Rob Jones brings in his 36-year-old wife because "one side of her face is drooping." Both anxiously express fear that she is having a stroke. When you question her, she tells you that she had a "strange pain" behind her right ear for a short time yesterday. This morning she noticed herself drooling out of the right side of her mouth when she brushed her teeth and drank her coffee. Her right eye feels "dry" and "it seems difficult to close my right upper eyelid." She denies headache, vision or hearing changes, or any other associated symptoms. She is normally healthy, has not recently been ill or experienced head trauma, and is on no medications regularly. She has no family history of cardiac disease or stroke. Your presumptive diagnosis for Mrs. Jones is:

    a. Cerebral hemorrhage
    b. Prodrome to herpes zoster
    c. Trigeminal neuralgia
    d. Bell's palsy

Questions 18 and 19 refer to the following scenario.

Mrs. Drew, a 62-year-old woman, presents for follow-up of her Parkinson's disease. She has been taking selegiline and benztropine for $1\frac{1}{2}$ years for the tremor in her right (dominant) hand. She lives alone and has been doing well. You have not seen her in six months because she went to Florida to stay with her sister during the winter. Today you notice that she moves more slowly, almost hesitantly, down the hall to your examination room. She tells you that she has noticed some tremor in her left hand in the "last few weeks," and "my writing seems to be getting smaller and smaller." She is feeling increasingly more fatigued, her "balance is off a little," and she has fallen twice since she got home.

18. Mrs. Drew's symptoms describe which of the following stages of severity on the Hoehn and Yahr Scale for the Severity of Parkinson's Disease?

    a. Stage II
    b. Stage III
    c. Stage IV
    d. Stage V

19. Typical of most patients with Parkinson's disease, during your examination you would expect to find that Mrs. Drew's deep tendon reflexes:

    a. Show no alteration from normal
    b. Are jerky and hyper-reflexive

c. Respond slowly and are hyporeflexive
d. Are erratic and vary with each visit

20. Which of the following antiseizure or antiepileptic drugs is the recommended first line treatment choice for absence (formerly petit mal) seizures?

a. Carbamazepine
b. Phenytoin
c. Valproic acid
d. Primidone

21. Most of the following general statements about treatment for seizure disorders are inaccurate or false. Which one of these statements is true and would be recommended in seizure disorder management/treatment?

a. Treatment of choice for recurrent seizures is usually a combination of two or three anticonvulsant drugs, depending on seizure type
b. Prophylactic anticonvulsant drug treatment is recommended for patients who have had only one seizure, even before the full diagnostic work-up is complete
c. If one anticonvulsant drug at high serum levels does not control the seizures, a second drug should be added to the treatment regimen, while slowly withdrawing the first drug
d. When a patient has been seizure free for one year, withdrawal of anticonvulsant medications should be considered; dose reduction should be gradual, over a period of weeks

22. Which of the following vitamins must be supplemented, in order to treat the signs and symptoms of Wernicke-Korsakoff syndrome?

a. Niacin
b. Vitamin A
c. Vitamin C
d. Thiamine

Answers and Rationale

1. **(c)** This patient's signs and symptoms describe the classic presentation of cluster headache. They occur in middle-aged men, are characterized by severe unilateral periorbital pain daily for several weeks, and are often accompanied by ipsilateral nasal congestion, rhinorrhea, and/or lacrimation. Episodes usually occur at night, awaken the patient, and last for less than two hours. Alcohol can be a trigger (Goroll, et al., p. 823; Tierney, et al., pp. 917-918; Wells, et al., pp. 647-648; Weinstock & Neides p. 131).

2. **(c)** Inhalation of 100% oxygen (a cerebral vasoconstrictor; usually prescribed at a rate of 6 to 8 L/min for no longer than 15 minutes) is one of the safe, effective alternatives for abortive therapy of cluster headaches. Ergot preparations, given either by subcutaneous injection dihydroergotamine (1 to 2 mg), or aerosol inhalation, and sumatriptan (6 mg), given by subcutaneous injection, are the other commonly used abortive treatments for cluster headaches. Oral drugs, (including oral sumatriptan) are generally inadequate or unsatisfactory for abortive treatment. Oral methysergide is used in prophylactic treatment of cluster headaches, as is lithium carbonate, and sometimes, corticosteroids, when the headaches are unresponsive to lithium or methysergide (Tierney, et al., pp. 917-918; Wells, et al., pp. 647-649).

3. **(b)** Vasodilation, excessive pulsation of branches of the external carotid artery, and neurogenic inflammation are the theorized causes of migraine. Current thinking is that vasoconstriction of branches of the internal carotid artery results in ischemia sufficient to cause the focal disturbances of neurologic function, including the aura, which precede or accompany the headaches, but not the headache pain (Wells, et al., p. 641; Tierney, et al., p. 916).

4. **(b)** Every item on the list of foods, stressors, and drugs in "b" is commonly listed as a possible trigger for headache; the other lists include none or only one possible trigger (Berman, et al., p. 58; Tierney, et al., pp. 916-917; Wells, et al., p. 642).

5. **(c)** Sumatriptan is used as acute, abortive treatment, of migraine headaches, not for prophylactic treatment. Other commonly used abortive treatments include aspirin, NSAID, and ergotamine preparations. All of the other drugs listed in options "a," "b," and "d" are commonly used for prophylactic/

preventive treatment of migraines (Berman, et al, p. 63; Goroll, et al., p. 827; Tierney, et al., pp. 917-918; Wells, et al., 643-646).

6. **(d)** Giant cell arteritis (also called temporal or cranial arteritis) usually occurs in older patients (> 50 years), and is characterized by a dull, aching pain, often caused by inflammation in the temporal, vertebral, ophthalmic, and posterior ciliary arteries. Symptoms may include scalp tenderness (especially on hair combing), throat pain, jaw claudication, and fever (in 15% of cases) with chills and sweats (Goroll, et al., p. 823; Tierney, et al., p. 807).

7. **(b)** The most feared complication of temporal, or giant cell, arteritis is blindness, which can occur when arteritis leads to occlusion of the ophthalmic artery. Diplopia may precede visual impairment (Goroll, et al., p. 823; Tierney, et al., p. 807).

8. **(d)** The pain of trigeminal neuralgia (tic douloureux) is often described as a unilateral lancinating pain which commonly arises near one side of the mouth and shoots toward the ear, eye, or nostril on that side (Tierney, et al., p. 919; Goroll, et al., p. 176).

9. **(b)** At this point in this patient's presentation, we would have to say that he is having a transient ischemic attack. Only if his symptoms and signs lasted longer than 24 hours could we say that he has had a stroke (Goroll, et al., pp. 858-859; Wells, et al., p. 161).

10. **(a)** The demyelinating process in MS commonly causes plaques and scarring in the white matter of the brain and spinal cord which can be visualized on MRI (Goroll, et al., p. 863; Tierney, et al., p. 949).

11. **(c)** Initial presenting symptoms of multiple sclerosis include fatigue, weakness or paresthesias in a limb and visual changes, including diplopia. The other symptoms listed in ''a,'' ''b,'' and ''d'' usually develop in later stages as MS progresses (Goroll, et al., p. 861; Tierney, et al., p. 949).

12. **(c)** Testing the voice for hoarseness, the gag reflex, and the patient's ability to swallow assess the status of cranial nerve X, the vagus nerve (Julian, p. 197).

13. **(b)** In Bell's palsy the corneal reflex is decreased on the affected side; the patient can feel the sensation, but cannot/does not blink (Billue, p. 99; Goroll, et al., p. 876).

14. **(a)** Optimal medical treatment of transient ischemic attacks in patients under age 65 is aspirin (Goroll, et al., 861; Tierney, et al., p. 929; Weinstock & Neides, p. 103).

15. **(d)** Endarterectomy is indicated in a patient with recurrent TIA if arteriography demonstrates high grade (70-90%) stenosis of a carotid artery (Goroll, et al., p. 861; Stobo, et al., p. 848; Tierney, et al., p. 457).

16. **(b)** The signs and symptoms in option "b" are not consistent with the diagnosis of carpal tunnel syndrome. In carpal tunnel syndrome, the median nerve is compressed, so paresthesias caused by Tinel's test (tapping mid-volar wrist) should radiate into the first three fingers, not four and five as suggested (fingers 4 and 5 are innervated by the ulnar nerve). The other findings are all consistent with carpal tunnel syndrome (Mercier, pp. 101-103; Stobo, et al., p. 258; Tierney, et al., p. 788).

17. **(d)** Under the age of 50, Bell's palsy occurs more frequently in women than men. Onset of facial paralysis is usually sudden and acute. Facial paralysis is unilateral and often preceded or accompanied by pain in the ear. Drooling is a common symptom, as is weakness of the orbicularis muscle, leaving the cornea unprotected (Goroll, et al., pp. 875-876; Tierney, et al., p. 964).

18. **(b)** Mrs. Drew's symptoms describe stage III on the Hoehn and Yahr Scale for the Severity of Parkinson's Disease: Bilateral involvement with mild postural imbalance on examination or history of poor balance or falls; patient leads an independent life (Wells, et al., p. 671).

19. **(a)** The deep tendon reflexes in a patient with Parkinson's disease are usually normal (Tierney, et al., p. 944).

20. **(c)** Valproic acid, ethosuximide, and clonazepam can be used to treat absence seizures. Carbamazepine is not considered useful for their treatment (Goroll, et al., p. 852; Tierney, et al., p. 920).

21. **(c)** Option "c" is a general recommendation for managing medications to control seizures in patients with seizure disorders. Option "a" is not correct—generally, monotherapy is recommended to begin seizure treatment. In most patients with seizures of a single type, satisfactory control can be achieved with a single anticonvulsant. Treatment with more than two drugs is almost always unhelpful, unless the patient has seizures of different types. It is also generally not recommended that patients who have had only one seizure be treated prophylactically with antiseizure drugs, and guidelines suggest that patients should be seizure free for at least three years (2 to 4 years in some references) before withdrawal of antiseizure medications is considered. Withdrawal for all anticonvulsants should be gradual (Tierney, et al., p, 924; Wells, et al., pp. 629–630).

22. **(d)** Thiamine deficiency is the underlying cause of both Wernicke's disease and Korsakoff's psychosis, commonly seen in alcoholics, so thiamine replacement would be critical in the treatment of those two disorders. IV thiamine is often given early in the treatment of Wernicke's encephalopathy, in order to minimize damage from the disease The other B vitamins are also usually supplemented (Tierney, et al., p. 1017).

References

Berman, G. D., Saper, J. R., & Solomon, G. D. (1996). Chronic headache: Management strategies that make sense. *Patient Care, 30*(2), 54-66.

Billue, J. S. (1997). Bell's palsy: An update on idiopathic facial paralysis. *The Nurse Practitioner: The American Journal of Primary Health Care, 22*(8), 88-105.

Goroll, A. H., May, L. A., & Mulley, A. G. (1995). *Primary care medicine*, (3rd ed.). Philadelphia: J. B. Lippincott.

Julian, T. W. (1995). *Health assessment and physical examination.* Albany: Del Mar Publishers.

Mercier, L. R. (1995). *Practical orthopedics* (4th ed.). St. Louis: Mosby.

Stobo, J. D., Hellmann, D. B., Ladenson, P. W., Petty, B. G., & Traill, T. A. (Eds.). (1996). *The principles and practice of medicine* (23rd ed.). Stamford, CT: Appleton & Lange.

Tierney, Jr., L. M., McPhee, S. J., & Papadakis, M. A. (Eds.). (1998). *Current medical diagnosis and treatment* (37th ed.). Stamford, CT: Appleton & Lange.

Weinstock, M. B., & Neides, D. M. (1996). *The resident's guide to ambulatory care* (2nd ed.). Columbus, OH: Anadem Publishing.

Wells, B. G., DiPiro, J. T., Schwinghammer, T. L., & Hamilton, C. W. (1998). *Pharmacotherapy handbook.* Stamford, CT: Appleton & Lange.

Psychosocial Disorders

Carol Gemberling

Select one best answer to the following questions.

Questions 1, 2, and 3 refer to the following scenario.

Ms. Daly is a 27-year-old graduate student at the local university who reports feeling "sad and blue" more than she feels happy. She works full time as a waitress at a local pub and is carrying 12 graduate credits. She recently discovered her boyfriend with her best friend and is both shocked and angered by this event. She mentions that for the past three weeks, she has been calling in sick and missing a lot of school. She denies drug, alcohol or medication use, psychotic or manic behavior. She finds it harder and harder to get out of bed before noon and lacks interest in eating or outside activities.

1. This type of behavior is consistent with which of the following conditions?
    a. Bipolar disorder
    b. Depression
    c. Acute anxiety reaction
    d. Insomnia

2. The ANP continues to interview Ms. Daly. The next appropriate line of inquiry would be to:
    a. Obtain a review of symptoms of the gastrointestinal system to rule out diseases which may mimic her presenting symptoms
    b. Obtain a complete family history of diseases and conditions that might be similar to her presenting symptoms in order to uncover a causative diagnosis
    c. Inquire about her grades, satisfaction with her present job, and her relationship with friends to see if any of these areas may be the cause of her feelings

    d. Explore any cognitive symptoms she might be experiencing such as feelings of guilt or worthlessness, impaired concentration, and thoughts of death or suicide

3. Standardized tools assist health care providers in accurately diagnosing conditions which might not be clearly defined. Which of the following tools for evaluating depression would be of benefit in working with Ms. Daly in the clinical setting?

    a. Tinetti scale
    b. Folstein scale
    c. Beck's inventory
    d. Functional assessment

Questions 4 and 5 refer to the following scenario.

Ms. McCleary is a 20-year-old fashion designer who presents with complaints of vague anxiety and a mild, fine tremor. She does not associate these feelings with any particular situation, but does report that there are numerous deadlines at work. She had similar symptoms as an adolescent that resolved without treatment but now she would like help with this problem as it is interfering with her everyday life. She denies taking medications, or drug or alcohol abuse.

4. What is the next appropriate step in the clinical management of this young woman?

    a. Carefully rule out all potential diagnoses, no matter how rare, which may mimic the symptoms of generalized anxiety
    b. Initiate pharmacologic treatment for phobic anxiety and recommend a few days off of work to relax and unwind before returning
    c. Begin benzodiazepine anxiolytics for her chronic anxiety and consider initiating cognitive and behavioral treatments at the next visit
    d. Gather additional historical data to rule out hyperthyroidism, hypoglycemia, depressive symptoms or panic attacks

5. Follow-up care including cognitive and behavioral approaches are planned for Ms. McCleary. Which of the following statements best reflects the correct approach to initiating these treatment modalities?

    a. Instruct her that after she has obtained complete control of her anxiety with benziodiazepine therapy, she should consciously recall that peaceful feeling when she is around things that make her nervous

b. Teach her to focus on the specific thoughts associated with her symptoms and examine the irrational fears associated with thoughts during times of greatest distress

c. Suggest that she consider a glass of wine on a daily basis to help her unwind, and gain self-control and mastery over stressful events she is experiencing at work

d. Teach systematic tensing and relaxing of specific muscle groups to help build skill and self-confidence in dealing with stressful events

Questions 6, 7, and 8 refer to the following scenario.

Mr. Reeder is a 61-year-old gentleman who reports problems with sleep and resultant difficulty staying awake during the day. He works the day shift in a newspaper printing plant and denies any new stressors at work. His best friend at work told him about a new sleeping pill that has helped him get a good night's sleep.

6. Which of the following statements best reflects the next step you would take in managing this patient's insomnia?

a. Ask him to call his friend to see what pill he is taking so that you can decide if there are any contraindications to prescribing it in his case

b. Have him stop all morning caffeine containing substances immediately and avoid any over-the-counter cold preparations as these may aggravate the problem

c. Ask about specific symptoms associated with awakening, determine the type of insomnia, and whether onset was acute or insidious

d. Advise him to take more frequent naps at the end of the work day in order to catch up on sleep which he may have missed during the night

7. A more specific history from Mr. Reeder reveals that he has difficulty falling asleep, and if he does "doze off," he awakens more frequently than usual. What information would you give Mr. Reeder about normal changes in sleep associated with the aging process?

a. Normal age related sleep changes include less time in deep stages of sleep and more frequent awakenings

b. Sleep needs normally increase with aging due to cardiac and pulmonary changes

c. The elderly spend 50% of their sleep in the REM stage which is much more restorative

d. Most elderly need only 4 to 6 hours of sleep in order to feel refreshed the next day

8. When planning Mr. Reeder's care, what specific information is helpful in maximizing his ability to obtain adequate sleep naturally?

   a. Medications such as benzodiazepines are very useful in chronic insomnia and have few side effects as compared with other pharmacologic agents
   b. Antihistamines, antidepressants, and anxiolytics have a safe drug profile and may be useful in elderly clients with sleep distrubances
   c. Nonpharmacologic approaches should be encouraged and can improve sleep complaints in at least half of insomniacs
   d. In order to catch up on lost sleep, listen to your body and rest or sleep whenever you feel the need

9. Mr. Caldren was recently diagnosed with multiple sclerosis. He has noticed a steady decline in his physical condition and is worried that his physician may have made the wrong diagnosis. He is very distressed at the prospect of spending the rest of his life dependent on others for his daily care. He has not told his family, who live in another state, about his recent diagnosis. What is the top priority with regard to Mr. Caldren's care?

   a. Contacting his family so that they can provide the kind of social and physical support that Mr. Caldren will need in the very near future
   b. Not asking any sensitive questions or discussing the progression of his disease because that line of questioning might lead him to harm himself
   c. Assessing additional risk factors for suicide and reassuring him that many patients are grateful to have their unmentioned plan discovered
   d. Evaluating him for the presence of contraindications to immunosuppressive therapy

Questions 10 and 11 refer to the following scenario.

Mrs. Radcliff is a 54-year-old patient who has been seen in urgent care on multiple occasions for multiple vague gastrointestinal, neurologic, and sexual complaints. She makes frequent and intense requests for medical care and many unscheduled visits to multiple providers. She has undergone repetitive but unrevealing evaluations because her symptoms are out of proportion to objective findings.

10. Which of the following diagnosis is most likely?

    a. Somatization disorder
    b. Myofascial pain syndrome
    c. "Worried well"
    d. Psychosis

11. After a careful review of Mrs. Radcliff's medical file and after obtaining a thorough history of her present complaints, no further diagnostic or laborarory testing is ordered. Which of the following elements is not an appropriate part of the treatment plan for Mrs. Radcliff?

   a. Spend time convincing the patient that no physical disease is present
   b. Suggest and arrange for visits with only one care provider who will be responsible for her care
   c. Be careful to not overlook objective signs of medical illness and order tests when indicated
   d. Increase the patient's awareness that psychological factors may be playing a role in the patients symptomatology

12. Mrs. Clemens is a 78-year-old home bound patient. Her son and daughter-in-law, who live a few blocks away, look after her. After not visiting for three days, her son finds her sitting in her favorite chair, unkempt, with spoiled food scattered around the kitchen and dining room table. She doesn't appear ill or have any physical complaints, but she has been acting less interested in his visits and in caring for her cat, whose name she can't recall today. She denies any appetite changes, incontinence, fever, or cough. What is your next step in caring for Mrs. Clemens?

   a. Take her to the emergency room immediately because it is clear that she is suffering from an acute psychotic episode
   b. Evaluate her for Alzheimer's disease because of her memory loss, and admit her to a skilled nursing facility for closer observation
   c. Obtain a more detailed mood, behavior, and mental status history to more fully evaluate her for symptoms of depression vs. dementia
   d. No action is necessary because she feels that her son is being overprotective; she was just more interested in television than cleaning her kitchen

Questions 13, 14, 15, and 16 refer to the following scenario.

Mr. Collins is a high powered attorney who presents to your urgent care with complaints of dyspnea, palpitations, dizziness, tremors, sweating, nausea, and a choking sensation. He admits to having these symptoms before. He denies any chest pain or paresthesias. He states that the symptoms seem to be unrelated to any particular activity, but fear and discomfort are associated with these symptoms which happen at any time of the day or night. He has been experiencing these symptoms approximately twice weekly, but in the past these episodes only occurred once every two months and were very mild. He denies ever smoking, using illicit drugs or abusing alcohol.

13. What serious medical problems should be ruled out?

    a. Cardiovascular events including angina, pulmonary embolism, dysrhythmia, transient ischemic attack, near syncope, or seizures
    b. Foreign body in the right bronchus, hiatial hernia, diabetic ketoacidosis, and volvulus of the sigmoid colon
    c. Emphysema with acute bronchitis, adult respiratory distress syndrome, paranoia, or acute alcohol withdrawal
    d. Hypothyroidism, paroxysmal atrial tachycardia, fever of unknown origin, or chronic obstructive pulmonary disease

14. Mr. Collins' symptoms of hyperventilation syndrome are produced by ventilation in excess of metabolic requirements. The differential diagnosis includes physiologic causes of hyperventilation such as pneumonia, heart failure, or metabolic acidosis. The diagnosis of hyperventilation syndrome overlaps considerably with anxiety disorders, and their precise relationship is controversial. Which of the following cluster of symptoms is most often associated with hyperventilation syndrome as compared with other psychological conditions?

    a. Tremors and myalgia
    b. Tetany and carpopedal spasms
    c. Nervousness and sweating
    d. Flatulence and bloating

15. Upon the completion of Mr. Collins' history and careful evaluation of his symptoms, the diagnosis of panic disorder was made. Which of the following statements made by the ANP would be the most therapeutic?

    a. "Try to relax and deep breathe, and when you have succeeded in gaining control I will return to give you the results of my evaluation of your complaints"
    b. Assist the patient in "talking through" the attack by reminding himself that "I've been through this before and it is terribly unpleasant but not dangerous"
    c. Inform the patient that "it is impossible to perform all the necessary tests that would rule out underlying disease so you'll just have to take my word"
    d. Inform the patient that "your symptoms of anxiety and depression can be easily treated with anxiolytics which are not associated with tolerance or dependence"

16. During a follow-up visit with Mr. Collins, you consider further evaluation and

a more structured, quantifiable, psychological assessment. Which of the following statements best describes the benefits and/or problems associated with this type of evaluation?

a. The accuracy of testing instruments is based upon the ability of the patient to give accurate information
b. The Minnesota Multiphasic Personality Inventory (MMPI), a widely used pencil and paper test, can be administered and interpreted by any member of the office staff
c. Structured, quantitative, psychological assessment instruments are inaccurate, rarely time efficient, and do not add information that will aid in the therapeutic process
d. Standardized tests are only helpful in cases in which historical information is either not helpful or somewhat contradictory

Answers and Rationale

1. **(b)** Two to three percent of the U.S. population suffer from major depression with the first episode occurring in adolescence or early adulthood, peak prevalence in middle age, and declining prevalence in later years. Females are approximately twice as likely to be diagnosed according to clinical and community samples. The hallmarks of depression are pervasively sad mood and markedly diminished interest or pleasure in almost all activities. These are typically accompanied by physical symptoms such as weight or appetite change, increased or decreased sleep, motor agitation or retardation, and fatigue (Fihn & DeWitt, pp. 631-632).

2. **(d)** In addition to the physical symptoms, cognitive symptoms such as feelings of guilt or worthlessness, impaired concentration, and thoughts of death or suicide may be experienced. It would be helpful to discover any family history of psychiatric or mental health problems, and to rule out cardiac or endocrine problems that might produce similar symptoms. Gathering a complete family and social history, as well as assessing her support systems, may also be of value in order to decide if her symptoms are "reactive" or "endogenous" in nature. Most importantly, discovering if her current symptoms put her at risk for harming herself, or if she has planned such an event, is of utmost importance and requires careful consideration and questioning (Fihn & DeWitt, pp. 631-632, 643-648).

3. **(c)** Several pencil and paper screening questionnaires have demonstrated sensitivity (80%) and specificity (70%) similar to a psychiatric interview. No single one has been shown to be superior to another, but the Beck Depression Inventory has widespread use in the clinical setting. The Tinetti scale assesses gait and balance, and the Folstein Mini-Mental Status Examination is helpful with dementia (Fihn & DeWitt, pp. 631-632, 643-645).

4. **(d)** Anxiety may be a nonspecific response to various biologic, psychological, and social factors. Although anxiety in primary care medical patients may result from undiagnosed medical illnesses, clinicians should avoid exhaustive efforts to rule out all potential medical causes no matter how rare. The common considerations include withdrawal syndromes, medication side effects, and intoxication, which were not likely in this patient. Other medical considerations include hyperthyroidism, hypoglycemia, and hypoxia. It is also important to note whether or not depression, alcohol or drug abuse, phobias, or panic disorders are part of the clinical picture. Benzodiazepine

anxiolytics are useful for the management of short term situational anxiety but should be avoided in cases of chronic anxiety states. For patients with nonspecific anxiety, cognitive and behavioral approaches should be the primary treatments instituted alone or in combination with pharmacologic therapies (Fihn & DeWitt, pp. 632-634).

5. **(b)** Cognitive and behavioral approaches to anxiety management focus on the half conscious, often unreasonable thoughts associated with anxiety. Patients are asked to focus on the specific thoughts that occur during times of greatest distress, and to learn to examine irrational fears associated with anxiety. This will help patients gain a sense of calm and self control. Systematic relaxation techniques work best when the patient avoids thinking about the fearful thoughts. For patients with nonspecific anxiety, cognitive and behavioral approaches should be the primary treatment. All patients with generalized anxiety, even those with no pattern of substance abuse, should be advised to avoid all caffeine and alcohol. The short term anxiolytic effects of alcohol are often followed by withdrawal anxiety (Fihn & DeWitt, pp. 632-635).

6. **(c)** Obtaining a thorough sleep history from the patient (and bed partner) if possible, is the best way to begin a sleep assessment. Specific questions regarding symptoms associated with awakening such as pain, dyspnea, palpitations, nocturia, or nausea can direct the clinician to look for underlying causes amenable to treatment. Stimulants such as caffeine in the evening, nicotine within a half hour of retiring, or illicit drugs such as cocaine may be at fault. A thorough sleep assessment may uncover a treatable cause for the insomnia, and pharmacologic therapies may not be needed or only be necessary on a short term basis (Fihn & DeWitt, pp. 635-638).

7. **(a)** A gradual change in sleep needs and frequent awakenings are viewed with frustration by some elderly, and as an opportunity to have more time for activities by others. Older adults have a decrease in total sleep time and stage 4 sleep, with more frequent awakenings during the night. Some may need to compensate with rest periods during the day. Newborns spend 50% of their sleep time in REM sleep; this amount gradually decreases to approximately 25%. Most healthy adults spend 7 to 9 hours sleeping each day, although many require less than 6 hours and many require more than 9. Normal age related cardiac and pulmonary changes should not have an effect on sleep patterns, quality or duration (Barkaukas, et al., pp. 124-126)

8. **(c)** Behavioral and cognitive approaches can improve insomnia in a significant number of patients. Implementing behaviors conducive to sleep are helpful in preventing common causes of insomnia. Examples of nonconducive behaviors include an unfavorable sleep environment, irregular sleep schedules, excessive time in bed, excessive napping, and a noisy or too light bedroom environment. Other factors which interfere with quality sleep include watching television or reading in the bedroom, uncomfortable bedroom temperatures, and worry. Many patients have anxiety about their insomnia, or are unaware that high body temperatures, due to physical exercise or a hot bath close to the time one retires for the night, may actually interfere with sleep. Benzodiazepines have limited use in chronic insomnia but can be used selectively for short periods (< two weeks); they may cause oversedation and dependence. They must be used cautiously in the elderly, patients with renal and liver disease, and heavy smokers. They are contraindicated in alcoholism, sleep apnea, and pregnancy. Nonhypnotics such as antihistamines, low dose antidepressants, and anxiolytics have significant anticholinergic side effects that may interfere with ambulation or urination (Fihn & DeWitt, pp. 635-638).

9. **(c)** Risk factors for suicide include male gender, previous history of attempted suicide, debilitating medical illness such as cancer or HIV infection, family history of suicide, depression, psychosis, alcoholism and drug dependence, unemployment, and poor social support systems. Health care providers who are concerned with bringing up the issue of suicide for fear that they may encourage a patient should be reassured that patients may be grateful to have their plan discovered. The clinician must be aware that the patient's ability to contemplate and plan suicide increases as they become less depressed and as their energy level lifts enough to allow them to successfully carry out a suicide plan (Rucker, pp. 589-590).

10. **(a)** Somatization is broadly defined as emotional distress that is experienced and expressed as physical symptoms. Patients who somatize chronically make frequent requests for medical care and have "much doctoring, little curing." Somatization and related psychiatric disorders are neither diagnoses of exclusion nor confined to the "worried well." The severity of somatization varies from transient amplification of minor physical concerns during times of stress to adoption of illness as a pervasive and disabling lifestyle. The DSM-IV diagnostic criteria require the presence of four pain symptoms, two gastrointestinal, one sexual symptom, and one pseudoneurologic symptom from an extended list of possible symptoms. The symptoms

must have been present for several years and resulted in treatment seeking behavior or significant social or occupational impairment (Fihn & DeWitt, pp. 639-642; Rucker, pp. 602-605).

11. **(a)** Convincing yourself and the patient that no physical disease is present is rarely possible or useful. Continuity of care with a single provider who is caring is of value with patients who somatize their symptoms. Patients should be seen frequently, approximately once per month, visits should be brief and should focus on the specific symptoms with which the patient presents. A normal examination and appropriate diagnostic testing should be performed on any patient coming in with these specific presenting symptoms to avoid overlooking medical illnesses. This approach is psychologically therapeutic as the patient will believe that the provider is taking the symptoms seriously. If the provider can approach the patient's symptoms as expressions of emotional disturbance, increase the patient's understanding of the relationship between psychological factors and symptomatology, and refer the patient for psychiatric help as indicated, the provider will be able to establish a therapeutic alliance with the patient with a somatization disorder (Fihn & DeWitt, pp. 639-642; Rucker, pp. 602-605).

12. **(c)** It is sometimes difficult to differentiate dementia from depression. The first step is a careful history from the patient and her family with regards to memory and mood changes. Although depression can be related to memory loss and lack of interest, so can dementia. Dementia is the acquired global impairment of cognitive abilities of sufficient severity to affect normal function. It must be distinguished from the minor forgetfulness of old age, which is normal. She is not exhibiting any symptoms of acute psychosis nor can we diagnose her with Alzheimer's disease. These behaviors need attention and careful evaluation in order to help Mrs. Clemens maintain a high level of functioning (Cutler, pp. 465-467).

13. **(a)** Recognition of panic disorder may be difficult because physical symptoms are similar to some serious medical problems and demand diagnostic testing. Symptoms of panic may resemble symptoms of almost any paroxysmal neurologic or cardiovascular event. Even when a diagnosis of panic attack seems likely, potentially life threatening neurological or cardiovascular events should be ruled out with a thorough history and physical examination, and any additional diagnostic testing that the examiner feels is necessary (Fihn & DeWitt, pp. 652-654).

14. **(b)** All symptoms listed in answer choices "a" through "d" may be seen in anxious patients, but tetany and carpopedal spasms are most commonly seen with hyperventilation syndrome along with acute anxiety and dramatic hyperpnea. The lines between acute anxiety and hyperventilation syndrome are blurred, but patients whose symptoms of tetany and carpopedal spasm are resolved by rebreathing into a paper bag are more likely to be suffering from hyperventilation syndrome (Fihn & DeWitt, pp. 660-662).

15. **(b)** Cognitive and behavioral techniques can be very effective in reducing panic symptoms and limiting phobic avoidance. Patients can be taught to remind themselves that they have been able to cope with these unpleasant episodes in the past, and that they are capable of coping now. The most important educational message is that avoidance of feared situations reinforces anxiety. Actively confronting feared situations will significantly reduce anxiety symptoms. Some panic patients may feel more anxious with breathing or relaxation exercises, so be alert for this paradoxical response. Anxiolytics offer more immediate relief but may be associated with tolerance and dependence. Reassuring patients that their complaints are not caused by organic disease can be very reassuring and decrease anxiety (Fihn & DeWitt, pp. 652-654).

16. **(a)** Many instruments that are useful for psychological assessments are available and congruent with the *Diagnostic and Statistical Manual of Mental Disorders* (DSM IV). The patient's ability to give accurate information is vital for most (but not all) of the psychological assessment tools that are available today. The MMPI requires referral to a specialist trained in the administration and interpretation of the test results. Structured, quantitative, psychological assessment instruments are accurate and time efficient methods of gathering information to improve the diagnostic and therapeutic process. Psychological assessment is indicated when a psychological condition such as depression, anxiety, or post-traumatic stress might be present and interfere with a treatment regimen, interact with a disease process, or affect the provider/patient relationship. These tools are also helpful when evaluating cognitive, affective, and adaptive functioning in patients who have known or suspected cognitive impairment. These standardized tests also provide helpful information to assist in counseling and motivating patients to change to a healthier lifestyle (Fihn & DeWitt, pp. 658-659).

References

Barkaukas, V., Stoltenberg-Allen, K., Baumann, L. C., & Darling-Fisher, C. D. (1998). *Health and physical assessment*. St. Louis: Mosby.

Cutler, P. (1998). *Problem solving in clinical medicine: From data to diagnosis*. Baltimore: Williams & Wilkins.

Fihn, S., & DeWitt, D. (1998). *Outpatient medicine*. Philadelphia: W. B. Saunders.

Rucker, L. (1998). *Essentials of adult ambulatory care*. Baltimore: Williams & Wilkins.

Care of the Aging Adult

Carol Gemberling

Select one best answer to the following questions.

1. When health care providers use standard adult clinical evaluation criteria, the assessment of high prevalence geriatric conditions may result in a lower than expected rate of detection. Which of the following areas of assessment is not one of the classical 5 "I's" of gerontological assessment?

    a. Incapacitation
    b. Iatrogenic
    c. Instability
    d. Incontinence

2. Which of the following laboratory tests best represents a change which may be seen as a normal aging variant?

    a. Erythrocyte sedimentation rate is lower in the absence of any significant inflammatory cause
    b. Alkaline phosphatase may be slightly elevated in the absence of liver and bone disease
    c. Fasting, two hour, and three hour blood glucose levels are expected to be lower than younger adults
    d. No laboratory abnormalities are expected in the elderly unless disease processes are present

Questions 3, 4, 5, and 6 refer to the following scenario.

Mr. Atkinson, 75-years-old, admits that in the past he has not always taken the medications prescribed for him.

3. Which of the following actions will improve overall compliance and safety with his pharmacologic therapies?

    a. Discontinue any medications he has forgotten to take on a regular basis
    b. Add new medications that will be taken to improve his forgetfulness
    c. Stop all medications and only prescribe those you know he will take
    d. Review the reasons for drugs prescribed, costs, and simplify regimes

4. After careful review of Mr. Atkinson's medication regime you decide that there are several medications which are unnecessary or are very similar to others he is taking. He is not taking one of his medications because of untoward side effects; you decide to initiate another pharmacologic therapy in its place. Which of the following recommendations should be considered when prescribing medications to elderly clients?

    a. Initiate medications that should be taken q.i.d. to assure adequate therapeutic blood levels
    b. In order to prevent drug toxicity, start with a low dose and slowly increase dosage taken
    c. Begin pharmacologic agents which are most easily swallowed and will be taken regularly
    d. Let the patient decide which drugs he thinks are important and only prescribe those agents

5. After several follow-up visits with Mr. Atkinson, it becomes clear that he is unable to care for himself sufficiently in the home environment. His physical condition has remained stable. At a family meeting, it is decided that admission to a long term care facility is appropriate. Soon after his admission, the nurses note increased anxiety and confusion, paranoia, decreased trust, and isolation. Which of the following actions is the most appropriate response by the nurses in this situation?

    a. Understand that these behaviors are commonly seen as a part of relocation syndrome and that they may lead to an increased incidence of falls and decreased mobility
    b. Consult with a psychiatrist because Mr. Atkinson is experiencing a new neurological condition which warrants a complete evaluation
    c. Discuss these changes with members of the staff and provide soft restraints whenever his behavior warrants protecting himself and others from harm
    d. Increase or add an anxiolytic agent to his therapeutic regime in order to control his inappropriate and potentially dangerous behavior

6. After careful questioning, Mr. Atkinson reported a history of urinary incontinence which caused him to need to change his clothing at least once during the

day. Which of the following statements best reflects the initial clinical approach in the evaluation of incontinence in this patient?

    a. Refer Mr. Atkinson to a urologist for prompt evaluation and treatment of a renal stone or bladder cancer

    b. Perform a straight catheterization in order to obtain a clean catch specimen for culture and sensitivity

    c. Exclude all causes of transient incontinence such as cystitis, medication side effects, or fecal impaction

    d. Order a tricyclic antidepressant such as imipramine to control overflow stress incontinence

7. Older geriatric clients present diagnostic challenges which are unique to the elderly. Which of the following statements best reflects a challenge inherent to caring for the elderly?

    a. They may exaggerate and complain about their symptoms more than a similar patient of middle age

    b. They sometimes confuse the provider with their detailed stories and often dwell on the past rather than the present

    c. They often worry about the normal body symptoms they experience which may confuse the medical staff

    d. They frequently present with an atypical presentation which makes a diagnosis more difficult

8. A comprehensive evaluation of a geriatric client is somewhat different from the assessment performed on a younger client. Which of the following components of assessment is of particular importance in the elderly population?

    a. Developmental
    b. Functional
    c. Psychosocial
    d. Financial

Questions 9, 10, 11, and 12 relate to the following scenario.

Mrs. Thomson is a 75-year-old thin Caucasian female who is being admitted to a nursing home. Analysis of her history reveals a deficiency in total daily caloric intake. Her social isolation and fixed income have contributed to her undernutrition.

9. The diet of an elderly person is often low in:

    a. Carbohydrates

b. Fats
c. Complex carbohydrates
d. Protein

10. Upon review of systems Mrs. Thomson complains of joint stiffness and pain. Which of the following types of arthritis is most common in the elderly?

a. Rheumatoid arthritis
b. Septic arthritis
c. Osteoarthritis
d. Crystal induced arthritis

11. While performing a mental status evaluation of Mrs. Thomson you become aware of some specific areas of alteration or decline in her cognitive functioning. Which statement best describes the difference between delirium and dementia?

a. Delirium is associated with impaired consciousness and attention while dementia is associated with consciousness yet difficulty in concentrating
b. Dementia is a more acute condition of altered sensorium while delirium may take months to years to be noticed by others
c. Delirium is a long term, irreversible change in cognitive abilities while dementia may wax and wane and be completely reversible
d. Dementia and delirium are rarely seen concurrently in the same patient so underlying causes need to be determined

12. During a follow-up visit with Mrs. Thompson, she tells you that she has been feeling more tired than usual and is unable to perform some of the tasks that she normally performs with ease. In order to help Mrs. Thompson, the nurse will need to clearly understand the difference between fatigue and weakness. Which of the following statements best describes fatigue?

a. It is usually accompanied by decreased muscle strength in single tasks
b. It is a feeling of extreme exhaustion not preceded by extraordinary physical activity
c. It is often associated with one or more objective physical abnormalities of the neuromuscular system
d. It is a specific inability to accomplish necessary daily activities several days in a row

13. Mr. Palmer is a 84-year-old patient who has been a widower for the past five

years and is showing an increased problem with urinary incontinence. He reports that his involuntary loss of urine is associated with the sensation of a desire to urinate, bladder spasms, and not having enough time to get to the bathroom. Which type of incontinence is Mr. Palmer most likely experiencing?

    a. Functional
    b. Overflow
    c. Stress
    d. Urge

14. Which of the following is not an expected age associated sensory change?

    a. Sudden onset of anosmia
    b. Gradual onset of presbycusis
    c. Presbyopia in young elderly
    d. Gradual progression of ageusia

Answers and Rationale

1. **(a)** The "Five I's of geriatrics" are areas which are characterized by high prevalence in the geriatric population and are associated with a lower than expected rate of detection by standard clinical evaluations. These areas include intellectual impairment, immobility, instability, incontinence, and iatrogenic disease (Lonergan, p. 7).

2. **(b)** The following laboratory changes are influenced by old age: Arterial PaO_2 may be lowered by age related changes in perfusion and ventilation; serum creatinine may be low and disguise renal failure in muscle wasted older patients; alkaline phosphatase may be slightly elevated in the absence of liver and bone disease; erythrocyte sedimentation rate may be elevated in old age and therefore reduces the value of this test; blood glucose levels of fasting, two and three hour may be slightly elevated (Lonergan, p. 8).

3. **(d)** Approximately one third to one half of elderly patients do not comply with prescribed medication regimes due to poor physician-patient communication, impaired cognitive functioning, adverse medication effects, duplicate prescriptions, high cost, complicated, medication regimes, and the fact that the patient did not think the dosage was necessary (Rucker, pp. 26-28, 46).

4. **(b)** Cumulative side effects are one of the leading problems encountered in prescribing to the elderly. Due to physiologic changes seen in the metabolism and excretion of pharmacologic agents, the lowest possible starting and maintenance doses should be considered. Multi-drug therapies should be avoided whenever possible. Simplification of drug regimes, and seeking to regularly review with the patient the need for each therapeutic agent, will greatly enhance therapy (Lonergan, p. 44-45).

5. **(a)** Relocation of an elderly person, especially to a nursing home, is a drastic environmental change which has the potential to cause untoward behaviors, especially if the change is unexpected and sudden. Examples of these behaviors include acute confusion (or increased confusion) increased anxiety, psychotic syndromes (such as hallucinations), and decreased trust or paranoia. These behaviors contribute to negative health outcomes such as falls and decreased mobility. In some cases, relocation has been associated with mortality. More subtle changes that have been reported include isolation,

decreased interpersonal behavior, and passive behavior (Ignatavicius, p. 15).

6. **(c)** The initial approach to evaluating patients with incontinence should be to rule out transient causes of incontinence such as cystitis, atrophic vaginitis in women, acute retention, restricted mobility, fecal impaction, acute delirium, or adverse drug effects which are most commonly caused by alpha adrenergic agents, anticholinergics, sedatives, narcotics and diuretics (Fihn & DeWitt, pp. 574-578).

7. **(d)** Illness in the elderly may be very confusing because it often presents with symptoms such as falls, incontinence, acute confusion, or failure to thrive when the etiology of the presenting symptoms is completely unrelated. When symptom onset is acute, reversible causes should be considered (drugs, common acute illnesses, or psychosocial problems) (Sloan, p. 153).

8. **(b)** The various components of the physical examination and health history provide an implicit indication of self care and overall functional abilities, but this may be insufficient in providing adequate information regarding the client's capabilities and activities. Functional assessment parameters can be integrated into a client's health assessment. If time permits, such integration can be highly individualized and provide health care providers with reliable data in order to make appropriate interventions for vulnerable populations (Barkaukas, pp. 713-714).

9. **(d)** Protein-calorie malnutrition is found in 30% to 50% of elderly individuals who live in nursing homes and hospitals. Borderline protein-calorie malnutrition is common in elderly outpatients. Multiple studies have demonstrated that elderly individuals commonly consume less than two thirds of the recommended daily allowance for multiple nutrients (Forciea & Lavizzo-Mourey, p. 73).

10. **(c)** The most frequent musculoskeletal condition diagnosed among persons over the age of 60 is osteoarthritis. Both upper and lower extremity impairments occur with increasing frequency in both sexes over age of 80 (Forciea & Lavizzo-Mourey, p. 38).

11. **(a)** Delirium involves a disturbance in consciousness associated with impaired

attention. This may manifest clinically as waxing and waning lethargy or diminished arousability, with or without periods of agitation. Patients with dementia are consistently arousable and able to remain alert without alterations in their level of consciousness; they may experience difficulty concentrating on a task and periods of agitation. An acute onset of confusion (minutes to hours or days) should always suggest delirium. Dementia usually begins insidiously and becomes apparent over a period of weeks, months, or years without dramatic improvement in cognitive or perceptual abilities (Forciea & Lavizzo-Mourey, p. 7).

12. **(b)** Fatigue and weakness are often used interchangeably, but fatigue is extreme exhaustion without a preceding, unusually strenuous energy expenditure. There is a generalized inability to accomplish necessary daily activities which may be due to difficulty concentrating on physical and mental tasks. Weakness is usually accompanied by decreased muscle strength in single tasks, reduced endurance in repetitive muscle activity, and one or more objective, physical, neurologic abnormalities (Forciea & Lavizzo-Mourey, p. 13).

13. **(d)** This is a very typical presentation of urge incontinence. Neurologic problems are often associated with this type of incontinence including stroke, dementia, Parkinson's disease, and spinal cord injury. Overflow incontinence is associated with incomplete bladder emptying, overdistention, and resultant leakage of urine without the sensation or bladder fullness; prostate enlargement, diabetes, and multiple sclerosis are common causes. Stress incontinence is an involuntary loss of urine when intra-abdominal pressure increases, as it does during coughing, sneezing or exercising; this is commonly due to relaxation of pelvic floor musculature. Functional incontinence is an involuntary loss of urine secondary to factors outside the lower urinary tract such as dementia, severe musculoskeletal problems, or environmental factors which make access to the bathroom difficult (Forciea & Lavizzo-Mourey, p. 186).

14. **(a)** Major changes seen as a normal part of aging include the gradual alteration of the sense of smell (anosomia). Sudden onset may be associated with a brain lesion. Presbycusis is a bilateral sensorineural, high frequency hearing loss which is commonly seen in elderly clients. Presbyopia, the loss of accommodative ability, occurs due to a hardening of the lens nucleus and ciliary muscle atrophy. Ageusia is the loss of sense of taste (Forciea & Lavizzo-Mourey, pp. 89-92).

References

Barkaukas, V., Stoltenberg-Allen, K., Baumann, L. C., & Darling-Fisher, C. D. (1998). *Health and physical assessment*. St. Louis: Mosby

Fihn, S., & DeWitt, D. (1998). *Outpatient medicine*. Philadelphia: W. B. Saunders.

Forciea, M., & Lavizzo-Mourey, R. (1996). *Geriatric secrets*. Philadelphia: Hanley & Belfus.

Ignatavicius, D. (1998). *Introduction to long term care nursing: Principles and practice*. Philadelphia: W. B. Saunders.

Lonergan, E. (1996). *Geriatrics: A Lange clinical manual*. Stamford CT: Appleton & Lange

Rucker, L. (1998). *Essentials of adult ambulatory care*. Baltimore: Williams & Wilkins.

Sloan, J. P. (1997). *Protocols in primary care geriatrics*. NY: Springer-Verlag.

Health Policy

Carol Gemberling

Select one best answer to the following questions.

1. The historical development of the advanced practice registered nurse (APRN) was fraught with barriers and obstacles which may have temporarily impacted their development and evolution. Which one of the following barriers was not an obstacle experienced by the profession?

    a. The rapid expansion of the role
    b. Medicine and pharmacy control issues
    c. Threatened liability coverage
    d. Lack of intraprofessional nursing support

2. Advanced practice nursing is divided into primary criteria or qualifications as well as core competencies which must be met before one can be considered an APRN. Which of the following primary criteria best reflects the necessary element for APRN practice?

    a. An earned master's or higher nursing degree
    b. Professional advanced level specialty practice
    c. Practice focused on patients and their families
    d. Advanced clinical nursing practice and knowledge base

3. Which of the following statements best reflects the necessity of change agent skills and knowledge for the advanced practice nurse?

    a. Change agent skills are essential elements necessary in order to effect change in clinical and organizational environments and to model these processes and skills for nurses in basic practice
    b. Change agent skills and role theory are a basic component of all APRN formal educational curricula in advanced practice nursing programs
    c. Change must be a necessary part of clinical practice skills and knowledge in order to convince patients of changes they must make for their health and well being

    d. Clinical nurse specialists and nurse midwives need change agent skills and knowledge more than other advanced practice nurses because of the settings in which they generally practice

4. The blended APRN role has been seen by some as an attempt to combine roles that are distinctly different in scope of practice. Which of the following statements best depicts the key benefit of blended role preparation of the clinical nurse specialist and the nurse practitioner?

    a. Blended role preparation provides a greater opportunity for nurse practitioners to provide a more in depth level of care to increasing numbers of critically ill patients

    b. Role blending would create a nurse who is uniquely qualified to provide a continuum of care which enhances continuity

    c. There would be a clearer method of identifying the advanced practice nurse's scope of practice by having a more simplified titling and definition of nursing practice that applies to the APRN

    d. A blended role curriculum would be easier to teach because all students would be essentially learning the same content in their advanced practice nursing programs

5. Accrediting bodies and administrators want evidence that the care delivery system will substantially improve patient care and contain costs. Which of the following statements best describes guidelines for differentiating research from quality improvement?

    a. Quality improvement involves data gathering intended to evaluate existing standards

    b. Quality improvement asks a new question that will expand knowledge with some generalizability

    c. Quality improvement frequently involves a risk to subjects that may be a part of the project

    d. Quality improvement involves the initiation of a new therapy or program as compared with standard approaches

6. Ethical decision making is an integral part of the role of the advanced practice nurse and requires considerable skills and knowledge in order to be effective. In order to function as an effective ethical decision maker an APRN should have:

    a. A working knowledge of the health care hierarchy and network with persons of influence in the setting in which she practices

b. Expert clinical knowledge and skill in order to be fully informed of the patient's options for care

c. Advanced knowledge of the history of ethics and ethical theories relevent to health care

d. Skill in problem identification, values clarification, negotiation, collaboration, and evaluation

7. The APRN as a case manager utilizes knowledge and skills which are inherent to all nurses in advanced practice. Which one of the following statements best reflects one of the key differences between the advanced nursing practice case manager and other APRN?

a. Advanced nursing practice case managers are required to have a master's degree and be certified as a case manager before they may perform any case management function

b. Advanced nursing practice case managers are less able to advocate effectively for the patient experiencing catastrophic illness

c. Advanced nursing practice case managers' accountability for accomplishing clinical, fiscal, and organizational outcomes is of greater importance than it would be for another APRN

d. The APRN is more likely to perform a more detailed assessment of environmental, organizational, and contextual factors that affect individual patients than the advanced nursing practice case manager

8. Health care at local, State, and federal levels is rapidly changing and the APRN is at the cutting edge in being able to work with policy makers and regulators to effect change. Nursing's involvement in the health care delivery system can help to solve the problems which are driving the need for health care reform. Which of the following best describes the areas where nursing can have the greatest impact on improving care across the nation?

a. Restructuring APRN education to include information on businesses and involvement in managed care plans as primary care providers

b. Improving access and primary care to the underserved, and restructuring hospitals and the role of public health

c. Improvement of health care service to poor women and closer monitoring of costs for health care to the elderly including end of life care decisions

d. Increasing APRN numbers in the work force, and overcoming barriers to care provided by the APRN in the hospital setting

9. The future of the APRN within the health care system is filled with turbulence and change. Which of the following is the most important attribute which will

enable the APRN to survive the dramatic changes seen in the present health care delivery system?

    a. Communication
    b. Caring
    c. Clinical competence
    d. Business acumen

10. Providing quality care, while keeping costs down, has been a difficult balancing act. Which of the following statements most accurately reflects the present state of affairs in providing quality health care services?

    a. Big corporations are waiting to see which health plans their employees are selecting before they renew their health contracts
    b. The National Committee on Quality Assurance is measuring preventive health care services provided in primary care settings
    c. Managed care organizations are more concerned with the evaluation and measurement of quality measures than they are with cost expenditures
    d. Medicare and Medicaid managed care organizations have the newest and most widely utilized measures of quality

11. Nursing faces many economic challenges in the 21st century. Which of the following do not represent challenges to the future well being of nurses?

    a. Adopting uniform licensure and educational requirements along with fewer and simpler titles
    b. Continuing to demonstrate that nurses are cost effective and provide high quality care
    c. Overcoming the mentality of an oppressed minority and sustaining a commitment to lifelong professional learning
    d. Viewing all nurses as performing the same roles and functions within the profession of nursing

12. Millions of Americans are uninsured or underinsured with regard to health care coverage. Which of the following statements accurately represents the current situation encountered by these American families?

    a. Many people choose to be uninsured and prefer to use urgent care when needed
    b. The uninsured get the health care they need from hospitals which provide charity care
    c. Being uninsured is a temporary situation for most individuals and doesn't last for more than a few months

    d. Uninsured statistics are in sharp contrast to coverage seen in other developed countries

13. In Barbara Safriet's seminal monograph, several suggestions were made to remove practice constraints under which the APRN must practice. Which of the following changes are needed by States in order to enhance APRN practice?

    a. Broaden nurse practice acts to include specific knowledge and a basic definition of an APRN, but not specific categories of APRN providers

    b. Encourage statutory requirements that promulgate the idea of supervision so that APRN malpractice liability will be minimal

    c. Maintain geographic and setting specifications so that the APRN will be able to practice utilizing standards within their community

    d. Continue to encourage mixed regulatory agencies control of APRN practice in order to maintain the highest standards or care

Answers and Rationale

1. **(a)** Inter and intraprofessional relationships surrounding the NP role present legal, legislative, and role issues which impact the control, regulation and development of the advanced practice nurse. In 1986, insurance carriers threatened to drop coverage or dramatically increase rates. National organizations were able to demonstrate the low risk nature of advanced practice nurses and this obstacle was averted. The APRN role has steadily expanded and the numbers of APRN have slowly increased. This expansion has not presented a barrier to the practice of the professional nurse (Hamric, et al., pp. 81-95).

2. **(a)** The advanced practice nurse must possess an earned graduate degree (master's or doctorate) with a concentration in an APRN category. The APRN engages in a practice focused on patients and their families. The term advanced nursing practice should describe advanced clinical practice (Hamric, et al., pp. 48-50).

3. **(a)** All advanced practice nurses need to be formally educated on change theory, strategies for change, and personal traits that enhance one's commitment to make change. Clearly, not all programs address these content areas in formal course work. These change agent skills can serve as a helpful modality in working with patients to make their own decisions about care choices. The APRN armed with change agent skills and knowledge can effect necessary and important changes in clinical and organizational environments as well as provide role modeling for other nurses (Hamric, et al., pp. 249-270).

4. **(b)** The blended role of the APRN integrates the CNS's skill of in depth assessment, and the interpersonal, coaching, and teaching expertise of both the CNS and NP into clinical problem solving and decision making. As a result, traditional medical evaluations and treatments are transformed, reflecting a synthesis of medicine and advanced nursing practice. The most exciting opportunity the blended role offers is to provide expanded services to patients, some traditionally considered within medicine's purview but now offered by the APRN who brings a nursing perspective (Hamric, et al., pp. 375-393).

5. **(a)** Research and quality improvement are different in that research may involve a potential risk to subjects, a new question may ask what will improve or expand knowledge, or a new therapy, program, or practice may be evaluated. In addition, research subjects' involvement changes their relationship with the caregiver in terms of patient care. Quality improvement offers a change in therapy, delivery of a new program, or the practice of an extension of standard care modalities. Monitoring patient or staff satisfaction with a new program as compared with existing practice, or the use of a measurement tool commonly used in clinical practice, is more a part of quality improvement. In addition, quality improvement involves data gathering intended to confirm existing standards, develop a new program, or refine an existing one (Hamric, et al., pp. 185-208).

6. **(d)** Ethical decision making skills are an art not a science. The APRN is in a key position to assume a more decisive role in managing the resolution of moral issues. Even though all of the choices could be of help to the APRN involved with ethical decision making, the skills of problem identification, values clarification, negotiation, collaboration, and evaluation empower the APRN to critically analyze and direct the decision making process. Being able to identify ethical dilemmas commonly seen in clinical practice settings, and realizing that the APRN takes on a more system wide vs. an individual patient approach to ethical dilemmas, can assist the APRN to engage in preventative strategies to improve ethical qualities of patient care (Hamric, et al., pp. 274-293).

7. **(c)** Even though there is considerable overlapping of functions seen with the APRN and advanced nursing practice case manager, the key difference between them lies with the case manager's accountability for accomplishing clinical, fiscal, and organizational outcomes. Case managers are frequently prepared at the baccalaureate level and certification is highly desirable. Advanced nursing practice case managers are generally in a better position to advocate for the patient in the area of attainment of goods and services that might be needed by long term, high use patients under their care (Hamric, et al., pp. 446-456).

8. **(b)** All of the answer choices contain some potential solutions to the present health care crisis. At the top of the list is our nation's need to provide more primary care services, and in particular more services to underserved populations. With the shift away from hospital oriented care, it becomes necessary to restructure hospitals and redesign the role that public health

plays in the provision of care. Finally, contributing to the viability of academic health centers will serve to insure a steady supply of primary care providers and support research efforts which contribute greatly to new developments in the provision of quality health care (Hamric, et al., pp. 497-514).

9. **(c)** All of the answer choices contain elements that would be of benefit to the APRN in her quest to survive system and professional turbulence. The most critical of the attributes is clinical competence. Additional attributes include caring, communication skills, business acumen and flexibility. These skills and attributes are essential for the success of APRN during these turbulent times (Hamric, et al., pp. 602-618).

10. **(b)** Quality measurement systems for managed care organizations at best lack clarity and recency. The administration of big corporations are selecting health plans based upon "value" and offering the best value to their employees. Medicare and Medicaid quality measures of managed care are at best antiquated and cumbersome. Managed care organizations have traditionally been more cost oriented (Harrington & Estes, pp. 210-242)

11. **(d)** Many challenges exist for nurses in the 21st century including uniformity in educational requirements and titling. Continued efforts are needed to confirm the quality and cost effectiveness of care provided. Learning to overcome job insecurity as the health care venue changes, and seeking to reinvent the nursing role by lifelong learning, are responses necessary to meet the demands seen in the health care marketplace. Finally, overcoming the mentality of an oppressed minority by assuming leadership roles within the profession, as well as in administration and government, is a challenge faced by the APRN (Harrington & Estes, pp. 164-172).

12. **(d)** All of the statements listed, except the last one, are reasons given to rationalize the large number of Americans who lack health care insurance. When the statistics are carefully evaluated, the numbers of individuals and families who lack health coverage is staggering. When care is needed, delays in seeking treatment are seen, and free or low cost care is inaccessible to many. The state of being uninsured lasts more than a few months for millions of Americans and is commonly seen in individuals who work full time but are not offered health care coverage. Our uninsured statistics are

amongst the highest in developed countries of the world (Harrington & Estes, pp. 334-340).

13. **(a)** Several changes have been suggested at the state level, which will assist in removing APRN practice barriers. These include: (a) a broader nurse practice act which includes the basic definition of an APRN but not specific categories, (b) elimination of all references to mixed regulatory entities, that is limit the regulation of the APRN to one discipline, (c) vest sole government authority over the APRN with the Board of Registered Nursing, (d) use no qualifying language for diagnosis and treatment, (e) empower boards of nursing to promulgate rules for the APRN, (f) eliminate statutory requirements for supervision, (g) enact nondiscrimination clauses to reform Medicaid and Medicare, and (h) remove geographic and practice setting barriers to APN care (Hamric, et al., pp. 511-513).

References

Hamric, A., Spross, J., & Hanson, C. (1996). *Advanced nursing practice: An integrative approach*. Philadelphia: W. B. Saunders.

Harrington, C., & Estes, C., (1997). *Health policy and nursing: Crisis and reform in the U.S. health care delivery system*. Boston: Jones & Bartlett.

Health Leadership Associates
Nurse Practitioner Continuing Education
Programs

Analysis of the 12-lead ECG

This course is designed for advanced practice nurses. During this 8 hour course you will review cardiac electrophysiology, the cardiac cycle and cardiac muscle function as a basis for 12-lead ECG interpretation; analysis of dysrhythmia, conduction abnormalities, atrial abnormalities, ventricular hypertrophy, axis deviation, myocardial ischemia and myocardial infarction. A one hour practice workshop completes the program. A comprehensive course syllabus is included.

Pharmacology for Nurse Practitioners: A Comprehensive Review and Update

This 30 hour course is designed as a comprehensive presentation and review of pharmacology from the physiologic perspective. In addition to presenting the pharmacokinetics and pharmacodynamics of drugs (indications, contraindications, mechanisms of action, excretion and side effects profile) the corresponding body system physiology will be presented in a format that makes the pharmacology easy to understand and apply in clinical practice. A comprehensive course syllabus is included.

Suturing Review and Practice

This $2\frac{1}{2}$ hour course is designed for nurse practitioners who do not have significant suturing experience. Whether you have been taught but haven't practiced, or have never been taught at all, this program will introduce and reinforce skills that you have not had the opportunity to develop. A brief didactic session on wound assessment and preparation is followed by hands-on instruction and practice of the simple interrupted and vertical mattress techniques.

For information on these and other programs contact:
Health Leadership Associates, Inc.
P.O. Box 59153
Potomac, MD 20859
1-800-435-4775

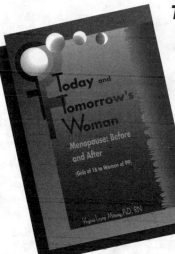

For information on Certification Review Courses, Home Study Programs and Review Books contact:

Health Leadership Associates, Inc.
Post Office Box 59153
Potomac, Maryland 20859

1-800-435-4775

REVIEW BOOK/AUDIO CASSETTE ORDER FORM
HEALTH LEADERSHIP ASSOCIATES, INC.

PLEASE PRINT OR TYPE

NAME: _____

ADDRESS: Street _____ Apt. # _____ City _____ State _____ Zip Code_____

TELEPHONE: _____ (HOME) _____ (WORK)

Section 1: AUDIO CASSETTES

Professional "live" audio recordings of Review Courses are approximately 15 hours in length unless otherwise noted and include detailed course handouts. Continuing Education contact hours are available for these audio cassette Home Study Programs.

QTY	REVIEW COURSE TITLE	PRICE	
___	Acute Care Nurse Practitioner	$150.00	
___	Adult Nurse Practitioner	$150.00	
___	Analysis of the 12-Lead ECG (Available 6/99)	$75.00	
___	** Childbearing Management	$ 45.00	
___	Clinical Specialist in Adult Psychiatric and Mental Health Nursing	$150.00	
___	Family Nurse Practitioner (Consists of ANP, PNP & Childbearing Management Courses)	$330.00	
___	* Gerontological Nurse	$ 75.00	
___	Gerontological Nurse Practitioner	$150.00	
___	Home Health Nurse	$150.00	
___	Inpatient Obstetric/Maternal Newborn/ Low Risk Neonatal/Perinatal Nurse	$150.00	
___	Medical-Surgical Nurse	$150.00	
___	** Menopause Lecture	$ 30.00	
___	Midwifery Review	$150.00	
___	* Pediatric Nurse	$ 75.00	
___	Pediatric Nurse Practitioner	$150.00	
___	Pharmacology Review and Update (Available 4/99)	$300.00	
___	* Psychiatric and Mental Health Nurse	$ 75.00	
___	** Test Taking Strategies and Techniques	$ 20.00	
___	Women's Health Care Nurse Practitioner	$150.00	

*8 Hour Course, ** 2 Hour Course

SUB TOTAL:		_____
Maryland Residents add 5% sales tax:		_____
CEU FEE ($25/course, except FNP course $35):	OPTIONAL	
Shipping: 2 Hour Course	$ 5.00	_____
All other Courses	$10.00	_____
TOTAL:		_____

PAYMENT DUE   METHOD OF PAYMENT

☐ Check or money order (US funds, payable to Health Leadership Associates, Inc.) A $25 fee will be charged on returned checks.

☐ Purchase Order is attached. P.O. # _____

☐ Please charge my: ☐ MasterCard ☐ Visa ☐ AMEX ☐ Discover

Credit Card# _____ Exp. date _____

Signature _____

Print Name _____

REVIEW GUIDES & AUDIO CASSETTES

1) Section 1 Total $ _____

2) Section 2 Total $ _____

3) Section 3 Total $ _____   (All prices subject to change without notice)

TOTAL PAYMENT DUE $ _____

Section 2: REVIEW BOOKS

QTY	BOOK TITLE	PRICE	
___	Adult Nurse Practitioner Certification Review Guide (third edition)	$ 47.75	_____
___	Family Nurse Practitioner Certification Review Guide Set (Includes ANP, PNP, and Women's Health Care NP Guides)	$123.25	_____
___	Gerontological Nursing Certification Review Guide for the Generalist, Clinical Specialist, and Nurse Practitioner (revised edition)	$ 47.75	_____
___	Pediatric Nurse Practitioner Certification Review Guide (third edition)	$ 47.75	_____
___	Psychiatric Certification Review Guide for the Generalist and Clinical Specialist in Adult, Child, and Adolescent Psychiatric and Mental Health Nursing (second edition)	$ 47.75	_____
___	Women's Health Care Nurse Practitioner Certification Review Guide	$ 47.75	_____
___	TODAY and TOMORROW'S WOMAN – MENOPAUSE: BEFORE AND AFTER (Girls of 16 to Women of 99)	$ 10.00	_____

STUDY QUESTION BOOKS

QTY	BOOK TITLE	PRICE	
___	Acute Care Nurse Practitioner Certification Study Question Book	$ 30.00	_____
___	Adult Nurse Practitioner Certification Study Question Book	$ 30.00	_____
___	Family Nurse Practitioner Certification Study Question Book Set (Includes ANP, PNP and WHCNP Study Question Books)	$ 60.00	_____
___	Pediatric Nurse Practitioner Certification Study Question Book	$ 30.00	_____
___	Women's Health Nurse Practitioner Certification Study Question Book	$ 30.00	_____

SUB TOTAL:		_____
Maryland Residents add 5% sales tax:		_____
CEU FEE ($20 per book, except FNP Set $35):	OPTIONAL	
Shipping: $9.00 FNP Set:		_____
$5.00 for one book:		_____
$2.00 for each additional book: (Except $1.00 for each add'l. *Today and Tomorrow's Woman*)		_____
TOTAL:		_____

For orders of 10 or greater call 1-800-435-4775.

Section 3: REVIEW BOOK/AUDIO CASSETTE DISCOUNT PACKAGES

A discounted rate is available when purchasing Review Book(s) and Audio Cassettes together. When purchasing packages, indicate Book/Audio Cassette selections in sections 1 and 2. *Does not apply to Study Question Books*. Calculate amount due in this section.

QTY	PACKAGE SELECTION	PRICE	
_____	8 Hour Course / 1 Review Guide	$120.00	_____
_____	15 Hour Course / 1 Review Guide	$190.00	_____
_____	FNP Package	$415.00	_____

FNP Package consists of Adult NP, Pediatric NP, Women's Health Care NP Guides & Audio Cassettes of the ANP, PNP, and Childbearing Management Courses.

SUB TOTAL:		_____
Maryland Residents add 5% sales tax:		_____
CEU Fee ($35 per package, except FNP Package $45)	OPTIONAL	
TOTAL: (Shipping charge included in package rate)		_____

RETURN POLICY

Due to the nature of the material contained in the review books and audio cassettes, returns on books ONLY will be accepted one week post delivery. No returns on audio cassettes except for defective audio cassettes which will be replaced.

MAIL TO:	Health Leadership Associates, Inc. P.O. Box 59153 Potomac, MD 20859
OR PHONE:	(800) 435-4775; (301) 983-2405
OR FAX:	(301) 983-2693

12/98

NOTES

NOTES

NOTES

NOTES

NOTES

NOTES

NOTES

NOTES

NOTES

NOTES